Avian Influenza or Bird Flu

Avian Influenza or Bird Flu

Dr. S. Nandi
Senior Scientist,
Centre for Animal Disease Research and Diagnosis
Indian Veterinary Research Institute
Izatnagar, U.P.

2009
DAYA PUBLISHING HOUSE
Delhi - 110 035

ISBN10 81-7035-595-8
ISBN13 978-81-7035-595-3

Published by : **Daya Publishing House**
1123/74, Deva Ram Park
Tri Nagar, Delhi - 110 035
Phone: 27383999
Fax: (011) 23260116
e-mail : dayabooks@vsnl.com
website : www.dayabooks.com

Showroom : 4760-61/23, Ansari Road, Darya Ganj,
New Delhi - 110 002
Phone: 23245578, 23244987

Laser Typesetting : **Classic Computer Services**
Delhi - 110 035

Printed at : **Chawla Offset Printers**
Delhi - 110 052

PRINTED IN INDIA

Preface

Influenza remains an important disease in humans, animals and birds. Avian influenza (AI) earlier known as fowl plaque or fowl pest, a highly contagious and infectious disease of birds, is now popularly known as avian flu or bird flu. All birds are thought to be vulnerable to avian influenza but poultry chicken, turkeys, quails, guinea fowls etc are more prone to AI virus which may reach rapidly to epidemic proportion. Influenza A viruses infecting poultry can be divided into two types: low pathogenicity avian influenza (LPAI) and highly pathogenic avian influenza (HPAI) or bird flu. Highly pathogenic AI has seriously affected poultry farmers whenever and wherever it has appeared. Historically, outbreaks of HPAI have occurred in all continents. Avian influenza virus is generally limited to poultry but an unprecedented epizootic of avian influenza A that is highly pathogenic has jumped the species barrier in Asia to cause many human fatalities and likely to pose an increasing pandemic threat. Zoonotic potential of AI virus was first recorded in 1997 with hospitalization of 18 people (six died) following the infection with HPAI (H5N1) in Hong Kong. On 18th February, 2006 HPAI virus infection in poultry has been reported in Maharashtra, Gujarat and Madhya Pradesh states of India for the first time followed by in July, 2007 in Manipur and 15th Janurary and 8th March, 2008 in W.B. Although the disease has been controlled in India, avian influenza is still prevalent in neighbouring countries and any moment it may enter into our country. Keeping in mind all the points, the book has been written on bird flu covering all the aspects in a simple and easily understandable manner. The book would be extremely helpful to the students, teachers, clinicians, technicians, researchers, farmers and general public. Lastly, comments and suggestions from all the corners are welcome to improve the quality of the book.

S. Nandi

Contents

1
Introduction

Poultry industry in India is a profitable industry which provide huge employment opportunity to a large section of the society. It is also the livelihood of many marginal and landless farmers. It is estimated that India maintains 1600 million broilers and 215 million layers in a year to produce 1.65 MMT of meat and 44 billion eggs. Globally, India ranked 4th in egg production and 5th in broiler production. This sector is growing at the rate of 8-15 per cent annually to contribute Rs 1300 crores to the national GDP. However, the poultry industry has been threatened by a number of infectious diseases of bacterial and viral origin and bird flu or avian influenza is the notable one. The consequences of the avian flu can be so devastating that it can wipe out much of the US $7.8 billion poultry industry. The recent outbreak of highly pathogenic avian influenza virus infection in poultry in Maharashtra, Gujarat and M.P. in

2006 resulted in the culling of over one million poultry birds, 1.5 million eggs and several thousand tones of feed resulting in huge economic losses of Rs 7000 crores (US $150 million). In 2007, Manipur Government culled 1.6 lakh domesticated fowls covering 5 Km radius following outbreak of bird flu (H5N1) in a private farm. The Government also provided compensation to the poultry owners to the tune of Rs 60 lakh for the purposes. On 15th January, 2008, bird flu outbreak has been reported in West Bengal and 16 out of 19 districts were affected. About 2.7 million birds were killed to contain the disease. Again, the disease reappeared on 8th March, 2008 in Murshidabad district followed by Malda districts of West Bengal. Bird flu in domestic and wild birds has been reported in 70 countries in four continents since it was first identified in Hong Kong in 1997. It has been confirmed in birds in China, Myanmar, Bangladesh, Pakistan and Afghanistan. China has confirmed three human cases and two deaths in 2007.

Influenza remains an important disease in humans, animals and birds. Avian influenza (AI) earlier known as fowl plague or fowl pest, a highly contagious and infectious disease of birds, is now popularly known as avian flu (AI) or bird flu. All birds are thought to be vulnerable to avian influenza but poultry chicken, turkeys, quails, guinea fowls etc are more prone to AI virus which may reach rapidly to epidemic proportion. Influenza A viruses infecting poultry can be divided into two distinct groups on the basis of their ability to cause disease: low pathogenicity avian influenza (LPAI) and highly pathogenic avian influenza (HPAI). The LPAI viruses cause only mild disease or asymptomatic infection whereas HPAI viruses cause systemic disease in poultry. The latter produces high mortality, resulting in significant economic losses. Over the last decades, highly virulent avian influenza viruses have caused outbreaks in poultry in various regions around the world. Influenza viruses have been shown to affect all types of domestic and captive birds in all the areas of the world. Avian influenza is generally limited to poultry and the frequency of primary infections in any type of birds depends on the degree of contact with the feral birds. Although viruses of relatively few subtype combinations have been isolated from mammalian species, all subtypes in most combinations, have been isolated from birds. In the twentieth century, the sudden emergence of antigenically different strains in humans termed "antigenic shift" has occurred on four occasions: 1918 (H1N1), 1957 (H2N2), 1968 (H3N2) and 1977 (H1N1) resulting in pandemics. An unprecedented epizootic of avian influenza A (H5N1) that is highly pathogenic has crossed the species barrier in Asia to cause many human fatalities and likely to pose an increasing pandemic threat. Zoonotic potential of AI virus was first recorded in 1997 with hospitalization of 18 people (six died) following the infection with HPAI (H5N1) in Hong Kong. Despite the presence of vaccines of proven efficacy, the influenza virus has developed avenues of counter assault that make vaccination a challenging and constantly changing task. In addition to its vast reservoirs, the influenza virus has alternative mechanisms to promote constant evolution and evasion of the hosts' immune response. The ability of influenza to undergo genetic changes in the form of antigenic shift and drift drives the continual emergence of antigenically and genetically novel viruses. The viruses resulting from the antigenic shift by the process of genetic reassortment are having the potential to cause the pandemics in humans. However, the Hong Kong incidence of human infections with the HPAI (H5N1) provided the evidence that HPAI strains of chicken can adapt, multiply and even cause death in affected individuals.

2

History

In May 1997, a young boy was died of viral pneumonia and multiorgan failure on the heels of an outbreak of highly pathogenic H5N1 avian influenza in chicken of farms in Hong Kong. The influenza H5N1 virus had been isolated from him in August, 1997. After all, it had been 29 years since the H3N2 pandemic virus was first isolated in Hong Kong in 1968. The region was subsequently recognized as a hypothetical epicenter for the emergence of pandemic influenza viruses.

Interestingly, the recognition of the index case of the so-called bird flu in early summer was at the time of the year hypothesized to be opportune for the interspecies transmission of avian influenza viruses to humans in the region. This is because of their greater abundance in domestic poultry particularly ducks. However, there were no further human H5N1 cases in the mid-summer months of June, July and August, when there is often much human influenza activity in Hong Kong, suggesting that the May case may have been a one off event. Nonetheless a state of alert was maintained.

In the mean time, evidence was emerging that all eight genes of the human H5N1 virus were of avian origin, the eight RNA segments of both viruses showing >99 per cent sequence homology. This indicated that the human virus had not undergone genetic reassortment with a prevailing human influenza A virus in a mammal, such as pig, the host or mixing vessel in which it was thought this would most likely occur. Such a virus is unlikely to produce a full blooded pandemic at the outset. In fact, a 4 years of regular surveillance in Hong Kong of pigs from China, the H5N1 virus was not isolated. It did not exclude the possibility that this reassortment could occur later in a human or that the virus could possibly adapt to humans through repeated contact.

3

Etiology

Influenza viruses are under the *Orthomyxoviridae* family and belong to either *Influenzavirus* A or *Influenzavirus* B or *Influenzavirus* C genus. The virus particles are enveloped with two types of glycoprotein projections having haemagglutinin (H) or neuraminidase (N) activity and contain 8 negative sense single stranded RNA. Influenza virions are typically spherical to pleomorphic but can be filamentous. Virions are 80-120 nm in diameter. The surface glycoprotein projections are 10-14 nm in length and 4-6 nm in diameter. The haemagglutinin peplomers are club shaped trimers and neuraminidase peplomers are mushroom shaped tetramers. Haemagglutinin is a type I glycoprotein (containing N terminal ectodomain and a C terminal anchor) while Neuraminidase is a type II glycoprotein (containing N terminal anchor and a C terminal ectodomain). The nucleocapsid is helical. Eight segments of single stranded negative sense RNA code for 8 structural and 2 non-structural proteins.

The haemagglutinin agglutinates RBCs and neuraminidase releases the virus from cells because of its sialidase activity. Two viral surface glycoproteins, H and N are encoded by the 4th and 6th viral segments respectively. Segments 7 and 8 encode two proteins each matrix 1 (M1) and matrix 2 (M2) and nonstructural 1 (NS1) and nonstructural 2 (NS2) respectively which execute regulatory functions in the viral life cycle. The minimum replication unit, a ribonucleoprotein (RNP) complex is composed of the viral RNA, NP (encoded by 5th segment) and 3 polymerase proteins (polymerase B2, B1 and A encoded by 3 largest segments). There are 16 haemagglutinin antigen (H1 to H16) and 9 neuraminidase antigens (N1 to N9) present in influenza A viruses. Each RNA strand of AI virus code for at least one protein. The H glycoprotein of influenza virus has two important functions which are imperative for the infectivity of the virus (*i*) it is responsible for attachment of the virus to the host cell receptors of glycoprotein or gangliosides containing sialic acid. (*ii*) it possesses fusion activity between the host cell membrane and the virus membrane so that virus genetic material is introduced into the host cell. The glycoprotein is produced as a precursor, HAo which requires post translational cleavage to HA1 and HA2, by host proteases before it is able to induce membrane fusion. Then only the virus particles becomes infectious. Type A viruses include the avian, swine, equine and human influenza A viruses. The large number of subtypes present in the type A influenza viruses are due to the fact that viruses often undergo antigenic shift by the process of genetic reassortment.

The antigenicity of influenza viruses changes gradually by point mutation (antigenic drift) or drastically by genetic reassortment (antigenic shift). Immunological pressure on H and N is thought to drive antigenic drift. Due to the changes in the antigenicity of human influenza virus, there is a need to replace the vaccine strains frequently. Antigenic drift has also been detected in avian influenza viruses but to a lesser extent than in human viruses possibly due to limited immunological pressure in short life span of birds. The influenza virus A type is most likely to cause epidemics and pandemics. This is because the influenza A virus can undergo antigenic shift and present a new immune target to susceptible people. The influenza B virus and C virus can undergo only antigenic drift and people are more resistant to these viruses as the new viruses have more similarity with previous strains. Antigenic drift results from point mutations in the genes coding for the viral haemagglutinin (H) and neuraminidase (N) due to infidelity of the viral encoded polymerase. Less frequent but potentially of far greater concern is the process of antigenic shift. Infection of a single cell by two different influenza viruses can result in the production of progeny viruses containing a mixture of RNA segments from the parental viruses. Reassortment between two different strains results in the periodic emergence of novel strain. It can occur between avian, swine, equine and human influenza A viruses. This type of reassortment can result in a 'hybrid virus', for example with virus proteins from avian and human influenza viruses. Antigenic shift is actually an abrupt change in the H and N proteins of influenza virus found in the host species.

Antigenic shift is caused by either direct transmission of non-human influenza viruses to humans or the reassortment of genes from two different influenza viruses that have infected a single cell. A total of 256 different combinations of RNA can be produced by reshuffling of the eight different genomic segments of the virus. Genetic reassortment is well documented both in vivo and in vitro under laboratory conditions. Mixed infections occur relatively frequently in nature and can lead to genetic reassortment. Reemergence of a previously circulating virus is another mechanism by which antigenic shift can occur. For example, the H1N1 Russian influenza virus which was circulating in the 1950s, subsequently reemerged in 1977 in human populations that were immunologically naïve to this subtype of virus, particularly younger persons, who had not been infected with H1N1 virus in the past.

HA also enables the virion to attach to cell surface sialyloligosaccharides and elicits virus neutralizing antibodies that are important in protection against infection. NA having receptor destroying enzyme (RDE) activity, aids in the release of the new virus from the infected cell, due to its action on the sialic acid cellular receptor thus helping the spread of infection. Both the HA and NA activities can be maintained even longer while the virus is no longer infectious. In addition to HA and NA a limited number of M2 proteins are integrated into the virions. They form tetramers, have H+ ion channel activity and facilitates the uncoating of the virus in endosomes at acidic pH. M1 is the most abundant protein lies within the envelope and thought to function in assembly and budding. Eight segments of ssRNA molecules contained within the viral envelope in association with NP and three subunits of viral polymerase

(PB1, PB2 and PA) form a ribonucleoprotein (RNP) complex that participates in RNA replication and transcription. NS2 protein now known to exist in virions is thought to play a role in the export of RNP from the nucleus through interaction with M1 protein. NS2 protein, the only non-structural protein of influenza A viruses has multiple functions including regulation of splicing and nuclear export of cellular mRNAs as well as stimulation of translation. It also counteracts the interferon activity of the hosts since an NS1, knockout virus was viable although it grew less efficiently than the parent virus in interferon nondefective cells. Beneath the lipid envelope there is a membrane or matrix (M) protein which surrounds a helical complex containing the nucleoprotein (NP) and polymerases (PB1, PB2 and PA) protein. There are also two non-structural proteins (NS1 and NS2) present in the virus. Each RNA strand of AI virus code for at least one protein. The H glycoprotein of influenza virus has two important functions which are imperative for the infectivity of the virus (*i*) it is responsible for attachment of the virus to the host cell receptors of glycoprotein or gangliosides containing sialic acid. (*ii*) it possesses fusion activity between the host cell membrane and the virus membrane so that virus genetic material is introduced into the host cell. The glycoprotein is produced as a precursor, HAo which requires post translational cleavage to HA1 and HA2, by host proteases before it is able to induce membrane fusion. Then only the virus particles becomes infectious. Type A viruses include the avian, swine, equine and human influenza A viruses. The large number of subtypes present in the type A influenza viruses are due to fact that viruses often undergo antigenic shift by the process of genetic reassortment.

Type B viruses are not categorized into subtype but are classified into strains. Influenza B viruses undergo antigenic drift by the process of point mutation but not antigenic shift commonly observed in influenza A viruses. Influenza B viruses can cause epidemics in human but not yet responsible for pandemics. Influenza B viruses cause disease in humans, ferrets and seals. However, these viruses have also been isolated from pigs and a horse. Serological evidence of infection has been found in pigs, dogs and horses. Influenza B viruses do not produce any disease in birds.

Influenza C viruses are not also classified into subtypes but are classified into strains. Reassortment does occur frequently between different strains of influenza C viruses. Type C viruses can cause mild disease in humans but have never been associated with large scale epidemics. Other than humans, influenza C viruses have been isolated from swine. These viruses can cause disease in experimentally infected dogs. Serological evidence of infection has been found in pigs, dogs and horses. Influenza C viruses also do not produce disease in birds.

Influenza viruses are composed of 70-75 per cent protein, 20-22 per cent lipids (phospholipids, cholesterol and glycolipid), 5-8 per cent carbohydrate (ribose, galactose, mannose, fructose and glucosamine) and 0.8–1 per cent RNA. The specific influenza virus isolates are identified by a standard nomenclature specifying the host of origin (excluding humans), geographical site of origin, strain number and year of isolation. The antigenic description of H and N is given last in parenthesis. Example A/chicken/Pennsylvanina/1370/83 (H5N2), A/Hong Kong/156/97 (H5N1).

The term 'superflu' is used to refer to a strain of flu virus that spreads unusually quickly, is unusually virulent, or is for which the host is unusually unresponsive to treatment. It is most commonly applied to strain which cause epidemics or pandemics. Virulence is a term used to refer either the relative pathogenicity or the relative ability to do damage to the host of an infectious agent. An epidemic disease is a disease that appear as new cases in the population in a period of time at a rate (the number of new cases in the population during a specified period of time is called the incidence rate) that substantially exceeds what is expected.

Details of the RNA and proteins of influenza A virus

Segment	*Protein Coded*	*Nos. of Amino Acids*	*Type*
1	PB1	759	Polymerase complex
2	PB2	757	Polymerase complex
3	PA	716	Polymerase complex
4	HA	566	Surface glycoprotein
5	NP	498	Protein associated with RNA
6	NA	454	Surface glycoprotein
7	Matrix 1 (M1)	252	Nonglycosylated protein beneath the envelope
	Matrix 2 (M2)	97	Integrated glycosylated membrane protein
8	Nonstructural 1 (NS1)	230	RNA binding protein
	Nonstructural 2 (NS2)	121	Nuclear export protein

Although viruses with all H and N subtypes are found in avian species, viral subtypes of mammalian influenza viruses are limited. Those which have circulated widely in humans are restricted to 3 H and 2 N subtypes (H1, H2 and H3 and N1 and N2 subtypes). Most of the human influenza A viruses are classified as H1N1, H2N2 (which circulated from 1957 to 1968 only) and H3N2. Pigs are susceptible to all subtypes of avian influenza viruses in experimental conditions but only the H1, H3 and N1 and N2 subtypes naturally. Two different subtypes of influenza A viruses (H7N7 and H3N8) have been isolated from horses, the former is commonly known as equine type 1 and the latter is known as equine type 2. Although both viruses produce similar disease signs in horses, infections caused by equine type 2 is more severe.

4

Pathogenesis

In poultry, the infection process begins by inhalation or ingestion of infectious AI virions. Because trypsin like enzymes in respiratory and intestinal epithelial cells allows the cleavage of the surface haemagglutin, multiple replication cycles occur in respiratory and intestinal tracts with release of infectious virions. In poultry, the nasal cavity is a major site of initial replication.

The replication of LPAI is limited to the respiratory or intestinal tracts. The illness and death is most often from respiratory damage especially if accompanied by secondary bacterial infections. Sometimes, the LPAI viruses spread systemically replicating and causing damage in kidney tubules, pancreatic acinar epithelium and other organs with epithelial cells having trypsin like enzyme.

HPAI viruses invade the submucosa to enter into the capillaries. The virus replicates within the endothelial cells.

The virus replicates within the endothelial cells and spread via the vascular or lymphatic systems to infect and replicate in a variety of cell types in visceral organs, brain and skin. The presence of haemagglutinin which is cleaved by furin like cellular enzyme is responsible for pantropic replication. Clinical signs and death are due to multiple organ failure. Damage caused by AI viruses is the result of one of three processes (1) direct virus replication in tissues and organs (2) indirect effect from cytokines and (3) ischemia from vascular thrombosis.

5

Receptor of Influenza Viruses

Although influenza A viruses uniformly recognize cell surface oligosaccharides with a terminal sialic acid, their receptor specificities vary. Most avian and equine influenza viruses preferentially bind to the N-acetylneuraminic acid alpha 2,3 galactose (NeuAcα2,3-Gal) linkages on sialyloligosaccharides, while human influenza viruses prefer the NeuAc α2,6-Gal linkage. Since avian and human influenza viruses show different receptor preferences, NeuAcα2,3-Gal versus NeuAcα2,6-Gal and epithelial cells lining of human trachea possess mainly the latter sialyloligosaccharide, it is considered that one of the determinants of the replicative potential of such viruses in different hosts might be the sialic acid-galactose linkage present on sialyloligosaccharides. A binding assay using two sialyloligosaccharide (NeuAcα2,3-Gal and NeuAcα2,6-Gal) specific lectins showed that the epithelial cells of duck intestine mainly contains NeuAcα2,3-Gal but not NeuAcα2,6-Gal, where as pig trachea contains both linkages. The lack of a suitable receptor accounts for the inefficient replication of human viruses in duck intestine and of avian viruses in humans. Moreover, detection of both linkages in pig trachea provides a molecular basis for efficient replication of human and avian influenza viruses in this host and hence genetic reassortment of these viruses.

With continued replication in pigs, we also found that the avian viruses appear to undergo a shift in their receptor specificity to NeuAcα2,6-Gal linkages exclusively. These observations suggest at least two mechanisms, both dependent on HA receptor interactions, that would permit pigs to serve as intermediate hosts for the generation of a hybrid strain with pandemic potential in a classical fashion. In the other, an avian virus would acquire the ability to bind efficiently to human cell surface receptors so that it could be readily transmitted to a human host without the requirement for genetic recombination. These models may not be mutually exclusive. Quite possibly, an avian virus could combine with a human virus before or after becoming adapted to the NeuAcα2,6-Gal linkage, resulting in a reassortant with enhanced proliferative capacity.

Although circumstantial evidence favors involvement of pigs in genetic reassortment, direct transmission of an avian virus to human does occur as exemplified by the recent incident in Hong Kong and the possibility of reassortment in humans or adaptation to recognize receptors in humans can not be discounted. With the rarity of human influenza pandemics, it is difficult to predict which of these models is more likely to generate a potentially hazardous virus.

6

Cytokines in the Pathogenesis of Influenza

Influenza A viruses cause severe epidemics of febrile respiratory illness in humans, horses and swine. Virus transmission readily occurs by the airborne route or by direct contact. In non-immune individuals, the virus multiplies rapidly in epithelial cells along the entire respiratory tract, whereas extrarespiratory spread of virus is extremely rare. Virus shedding and disease usually begin within 18-72 h after infection. The available data suggest that the lungs are even more susceptible than the upper respiratory tract, and very high titres (up to 10^9 50 per cent egg infectious doses EID_{50}/ml) have been recovered from fatal cases of human influenza pneumonia. Nasal and bronchial biopsy specimen reveal degeneration and desquamation of epithelial cells, and initially, a marked infiltration of neutrophils in the airways. These neutrophils play an important role in the pathophysiology of influenza as they cause narrowing of terminal bronchi/bronchioli and correlate with the onset of fever in experimental animal models. Characteristic clinical signs involve both the upper and lower respiratory tracts and include nasal obstruction and discharge, sore throat, cough and breathing difficulties. Fever, chill, headache, myalgias, malaise and anorexia are predominant symptoms. Degeneration of the respiratory tract epithelium and the onset of disease are extremely rapid, but regeneration with clinical recovery and viral clearance frequently occur within 7 days.

Despite extensive clinical and pathological descriptions of influenza, the mechanisms of disease development is still incomplete. There is, however, growing evidence that the so called early cytokines are the cause of many of the clinical signs. Early cytokines are produced by non immune cells at the site of infection and they are responsible for local inflammatory reactions, as well as some systemic effects. Interferon α, TNF α and IL-1 α and β theoretically stand most proximal in the early cytokine cascade. These cytokines are rapidly followed by IL-6 and a number of chemotactic cytokines, such as the neutrophil attracting IL-8, the macrophage inflammatory proteins and monocyte chemoattractant protein. IFN–α, TNF α, IL-1 and IL-6 are typical examples of cytokines with multifunctional activities and all of them have been associated with fever, excessive sleepiness and anorexia. TNF–α and IL-1 are well known for their profound stimulating effects on neutrophil and macrophage functions. Both cytokines strongly upregulate leukocyte adhesion molecules on the vascular endothelium, thereby mediating the first essential step for sequestration of neutrophils and or macrophages into the respiratory tract. True chemokines then give the signal for the directed migration of neutrophils or mesenteric macrophages into the tissues.

Many of these early response of cytokines have overlapping and synergistic activities and can even induce their own production or that of other cytokines. TNF–α and IL-1, for example, stimulate the release of IL-6 and some chemokines. Both the production and actions of cytokines are thus critically dependent on the context in which they occur.

7

Virus and the Disease

Influenza A viruses infecting poultry birds can be divided into two distinct groups on the basis of their ability to cause disease in chickens. The very virulent viruses called highly pathogenic avian influenza (HPAI) or bird flu in which mortality may be as high as 100 per cent. These viruses have been restricted to subtypes H5 and H7, although most of the viruses of these subtypes cause only low pathogenicity avian influenza (LPAI) and only a few percentages of all H5 and H7 subtypes of AI viruses cause HPAI. All the other subtypes of AI viruses have been reported in the majority of possible combinations from the birds and cause only LPAI. It is to be noted that the two H10 subtype (H10N4 and H10N5) of influenza A viruses have also been reported to be fulfilling the criteria given by OIE and EU of becoming the HPAI.

The HPAI can cause serious infections in some species of birds on a farm while leaving others unaffected. The clinical signs are variable. The typical symptoms are sinusitis, lacrymation, oedema of head, cyanosis of the head, comb and wattle and green to white diarrhea. Haemorrhagic lesions are observed on the comb and wattle of turkeys. Anorexia, coughing, sneezing, blood tinged oral and nasal discharge, ecchymoses on the shanks of feet, neurological symptoms and reduced egg production, loss of egg pigmentation and deformed or shell less eggs are also commonly observed signs. Sudden death may occur with other symptoms. Most of the flock usually die. In ducks, the most common symptoms are sinusitis, diarrhea and increased mortality.

The low pathogenic avian influenza (LPAI) viruses usually cause subclinical or mild illness. The symptoms may include decreased egg production, mild to moderate respiratory disease and low mortality rate (5 per cent). More severe disease mimicking highly pathogenic avian influenza with high mortality (up to 50 per cent) may also be seen in birds infected with LPAI when the condition is aggravated due to presence of secondary bacterial infection or other intercurrent viral diseases.

Most of the AI infections do not produce any recognizable disease in free living or wild birds. All these birds are the asymptomatic reservoirs of the AI viruses. Wild waterfowl and other aquatic birds (ducks, geese, shorebirds, gulls, swans, terns etc.) are the reservoir of all AI viruses. Natural infections of wild birds with HPAI are rare. Viruses of H5 or H7 subtypes isolated from the free living birds are almost invariably of low pathogenicity for poultry. Seasonal coming of migratory waterfowls may allow the regular addition of new viruses to the diverse domestic poultry virus pool in the backyard poultry system.

Lesions

HPAI in poultry birds may cause oedematous, haemorrhagic and necrotic lesions in skin and visceral organs namely lungs, spleen, heart, liver, kidney, pancreas etc. Petechial haemorrhages of whole viscera and peritoneum with generalized congestion are observed. Histologically, multiorgan necrosis and/or inflammation occurs. Brain, heart, lung and pancreas along with primary and secondary lymphoid organs are most severely affected. There is perivascular cuffing of lymphocytes in brain, heart, spleen and pancreas, coagulative necrosis in kidney, lungs and spleen, haemorrhagic streaks in heart muscles with focal degeneration to necrosis, urate casts in kidney tubules, lymphocytic meningoencephalitis with focal gliosis and neuronal necrosis. Necrosis, apoptosis and depletion of lymphocytes are common in the bursa, thymus and spleen.

LPAI in poultry birds may produce lesions in respiratory tract especially the sinusitis and tracheitis with thickened mucous and catarrhal, fibrinous and mucopurulent inflammation. The tracheal mucosa can be oedematous with congestion and haemorrhages. Microscopically there is diffused pneumonia, heterophilic to lymphocytic tracheitis and bronchitis, nephrosis and nephritis, pancreatitis, lymphocyte depletion and apoptosis of lymphocytes in the bursa, thymus and spleen.

8

Susceptibility to Physical and Chemical Agents

Avian influenza viruses are relatively unstable in the environment. Physical agents such as heat, extremes of pH, non-isotonic condition and dryness can inactivate avian influenza viruses. As avian influenza viruses are enveloped they are readily inactivated by organic solvents and detergents such as Na deoxycholate and SDS. In the presence of organic matter, AI virus can be destroyed by chemical inactivants such as aldehyde (HCHO or glutaraldehyde), betapropriolactone (BPL) and binary ethyleneimine (BEI). After removal of organic matter, chemical disinfectants such as phenolics, quaternary ammonium compound, oxidizing agent (Na hypochloride), acid and hydroxylamine can destroy AI viruses. Inactivation with retention of haemagglutinating and neuraminidase activities can be achieved with various concentration of formalin, BEI and BPL used as inactivants in vaccine production.

In the field condition, influenza viruses are protected by organic material such as nasal secretions or faeces which increase the resistance to physical and chemical inactivation. Cool and moist conditions favour long survival of AI viruses in the environment. AI viruses are viable in liquid manure for 105 days in the winter and in faeces for 35 days at 4°C and 7 days at 20°C.

Proper inactivation and elimination of AI viruses shed in the environment is essential in the control of field infections and can be accomplished by heating of building to 90-100°C, thorough removal and disposal of manure and litter, cleaning and disinfecting building and equipment and allowing 3 months vacancy period before restocking. Virus in the manure and litter must be inactivated and disposed of by burial, composting or incineration. Effective disinfectants clear surfaces are 5.25 per cent Na hypochloride, 2 per cent NaOH, strong oxidising ionophor compounds, chlorine dioxide, strong oxidising agents and 4 per cent Na_2CO_3 and 0.1 per cent Na silicate.

9

Ecology

Influenza A viruses have been detected in more than 90 species of apparently healthy wild birds. Wild waterfowl, gulls and shore birds are the natural reservoir of all influenza A viruses, without developing symptoms, for thousand of years in an environment that is optimal for adaptation of the virus to the host. These birds are highly mobile and wild waterfowl particularly are known to carry viruses over great distances and to excrete large quantities of viruses in their faeces while remaining perfectly healthy. After circulating for short periods of time in a poultry population, viruses of low pathogenicity can mutate into highly pathogenic viruses. An example was the H5N2 virus that circulated in the US in 1983 to 1984, beginning with a low mortality rate but within 6 months becoming highly pathogenic with a mortality rate approaching 90 per cent.

Another example was the epidemic in Italy of the H7N1 virus which began with low pathogenicity but mutated within 9 months of a highly pathogenic form, with more than 13 million birds dying or being put to death.

Influenza Viruses in Birds and Mammals

Influenza viruses can infect a wide variety of birds and mammals thus demonstrating an unusually wide host range. Influenzavirus appears to be well adapted to the natural host (wild aquatic birds) causing little or no disease. However, when influenza viruses infect non-host species, disease can often result. Serious disease outbreak have been reported for poultry species, primarily chickens and turkeys as well as mammals such as pigs, horses, mink, seals and humans. Although influenza viruses are considered to be pathogens adapted to a particular species, numerous exceptions have occurred. For example, classic H1N1 swine influenza viruses generally only infect pigs, but it has been known to infect humans and turkeys often causing serious disease. Avian influenza viruses have caused epizootics of respiratory disease in mink, seals and whales. A few cases of natural infections by AI viruses in humans have been reported. In experimental studies, AI viruses have been shown to infect pigs, ferrets, rats, rabbits, guinea pigs, mice, cats, mink, non-human primates and humans.

LPAI Viruses in Wild Birds

LPAI viruses are worldwide in distribution, predominantly infecting a variety of wild birds species but also some domestic birds. LPAI viruses have been isolated in wild birds from five continents including North America, Europe, Asia, Africa and Australia. Serological evidence has been reported in wild birds from Antarctica. Some AI infections have involved wild terrestrial birds but these birds do not represent a major source or reservoir of AI viruses. Briefly, AI viruses have been isolated from more than 90 species of free living birds representing 13 different orders: Anseriformes (ducks, geese and swans), Charadriiformes (turnstones, sandpipers, gulls, terns, puffins and guillemots), Ciconiiformes (herons and ibis), Columbiformes (doves), Falconiformes (raptors), Galliformes (partridge and pheasant), Gaviiformes (loons), Gruiformes (coots and moohen), Passeriformes (mynah, finch and weaver birds), Pelecaniformes (cormorant), Piciformes (woodpecker), Podicipediformes (grebe) and Procellariformes (shear water). This represents <1 per cent of known avian species, but the actual number of naturally infected species is most likely much greater. Most AI infection do not produce recognizable disease in free living birds.

In man made ecosystem, infections have been reported in Psittaciformes (parrorts, cockatoos and parakeets), Casuariiformes (emu), Struthioniformes (ostrich), Rheiformes (rhea) and domesticated Galliformes and Anseriformes. This latter two groups include chickens, turkeys, Japanese quail (*coturnix japonica*), helmeted guineafowl (*Numida meleagris*), Bobwhite quail (*Colinus virginianus*), pheasants, chukar partridges (*Alectoris chukar*), geese and ducks (mallards and muscovy).

Although influenza viruses can infect large numbers of wild waterfowl, infection usually only produces an asymptomatic enteric infection. Infected birds can produce large amount of virus often defecated directly into the water. The contamination of the aquatic environment appears to be an efficient method of transmission of virus to susceptible wild or domestic birds which share the same environment.

LPAI in Domestic Birds

Chickens and turkeys can be readily infected with AI virus.. The direct transmission of influenza viruses from migrating waterfowl to range-reared turkeys has been implicated as a common source of infection in the USA and probably also plays a major role in transmission of AI to chickens. The transmission of influenza from wild waterfowl to chickens and turkeys may also occur through domestic ducks and geese that are reared or marketed in close association with chickens and turkeys. Once influenza viruses have been introduced into commercial poultry operations the virus can spread to new locations and maintained for long periods of time. Additionally, LPAI viruses have been isolated from ducks, quail and game birds. Although AI infection in these birds may be asymptomatic, outbreaks of respiratory disease with mortality have been reported. AI viruses in poultry is transmitted through respiratory secretions and faeces.

HPAI Viruses

No wild bird reservoir has been identified for HPAI viruses. Except for the single outbreak of HPAI in common terns in South Africa, HPAI has been rarely isolated from wild birds even on farms experiencing outbreaks of HPAI in domestic poultry. In 1983-84 in Pennsylvania and 1994-95 in Mexico, avian influenza outbreaks showed that HPAI viruses arose following mutation of H5 LPAI which circulated widely in domestic poultry. An experimental chicken embryo model has shown that some H5 and H7 LPAI viruses can mutate to form HPAI viruses that are similar pathobiologically and molecularly to HPAI field virus. It suggests that HPAI viruses arise in domestic poultry population from LPAI viruses and are not widely maintained as HPAI in wild bird populations. However, small groups of wild birds serve as reservoirs of HPAI viruses derived from poultry.

10

Incidences and Distribution

AI viruses have a worldwide distribution with reports of isolations from Africa, Asia, Australia, Europe and North and South America and serological evidence of infection in penguin from Antarctica. The source of AI viruses has been free living aquatic birds especially of the orders Anseriformes (duck and geese) and Charadriiformes (shore birds, gulls, terns and auks) which are considered genetic reservoirs of all AI viruses. In these species AI virus infections cause little or no disease with the exception of high mortality in common terns in South Africa in 1961. AI viruses have been commonly isolated from all 11 North American species of pond and river ducks and H3, H4, H6, N2, N6 and N8 are readily isolated. Most combinations of the 16 H and 9 N subtypes are isolated from aquatic free living birds but infrequently from wild terrestrial birds.

Although influenza viruses can infect large number of wild waterfowl, infection usually only produces an asymptomatic enteric infection. Infected birds can produce large amount of virus often defecated directly into the water. The contamination of the aquatic environment appears to be an efficient method of transmission of virus to susceptible wild birds or to domestic birds which share the same environment. Water contaminated with AI virus in the faeces of infected wild ducks has been a source of infection for domestic turkey.

AI viruses have been isolated sporadically from domestic poultry, most frequently chickens, turkeys, ducks and captive birds. However, incidence and distribution varies greatly with geographical location, species, age of bird, time of year and environmental conditions. Turkeys and other gallinaceous birds (including chickens) are not natural reservoirs of AI viruses. Due to the alteration of the natural ecosystems of birds through captivity, domestication, industrial agriculture, national and international commerce by humans has created new niches for AI viruses and variations in the incidence and distribution of AI infections.

Most influenza infections in domestic poultry have been from avian origin influenza viruses. However, H1N1 and H1N2 swine influenza viruses have infected turkeys, especially turkey breeders, causing significant disease problems.

11

Incubation Period, Transmission and Epidemiology

Incubation Period

The incubation period varies from few hours in intravenously inoculated birds to 3 days in naturally infected individual birds and up to 14 days in a flock. The incubation period is dependent on the dose of virus, the route of exposure, the species exposed and the ability to detect clinical signs.

Transmission

As the virus is replicated in the respiratory, intestinal, and /or reproductive organs, AI virus is excreted from the nares, mouth, conjunctive and cloaca of infected birds. In intranasally inoculated 21 days old chickens peak level of HPAI virus from the oropharynx is $10^{4.2-7.7}$ EID_{50}/ml of respiratory secretions and from the cloaca $10^{2.5-4.5}$ EID_{50}/g of faeces. Avian influenza virus can persist for up to 2 weeks in faeces and on cages 32 days at 15-20°C and at least 20 days at 28-30°C. They can survive indefinitely when frozen.

Although virus is transmitted between infected and susceptible birds through direct contact or indirect contact through aerosol droplets or virus contaminated fomites. Aerosol transmission is a significant mode of transmission because of high virus concentration in the respiratory tract. AI viruses are readily transported to other premises by people and equipment shared in production and live bird marketing.

Influenza viruses exhibit varying degrees of adaptation to individual host species with frequent and easy intraspecies transmission. Interspecies transmission usually occur between closely related host species in the same taxonomic family such as turkeys, chickens, guineafowls and quail of the Order *Galliformes*, Family *Phasianidae*. Interspecies transmission can occur less frequently across different orders within same class such as from free flying duck (Order *Anseriformes*) to turkey (Order *Galliformes*). Furthermore interspecies transmission between different phylogenetic classes is even less frequent as occurred rarely with chicken to human. Many factors such as geographic restriction of host distribution, intermixing of species, age and density of birds, weather and temperature also play an important role in the transmission of AI viruses within and between host species.

As the source of infection for the initial introduction of the influenza virus into commercial poultry flocks include other domestic and confined poultry, migratory waterfowl, domestic pigs and companion or pet birds, producers should raise only one species of bird in an individual operation and add new birds only after testing and quarantine and practice high degree of biosecurity to minimize the risk of introduction and dissemination of AI viruses.

AI virus infection of hens has resulted in virus recovery from the egg shell surface and the internal content of the eggs. Cleaning of faecal material and disinfection of egg shells may be necessary to prevent the hatchery associated dissemination of AI virus. In experimental studies, AI virus has been shown to replicate and be excreted from individual ducks for up to 30 days, chickens for up to 36 days and turkeys for up to 72 days. However, on a population basis, AI virus can be maintained for much longer time periods in agricultural operations. Once a flock is infected, it should be considered a potential source of virus for life. In wild waterfowl, AI viruses are maintained by passage in susceptible birds throughout the year.

Epidemiology

Surveys indicate the presence of mostly benign low pathogenic avian influenza (LPAI) viruses of many known H and N subtypes in free ranging avian species, including migratory birds. Low pathogenic viruses can after circulation for some time in a poultry populations, mutate into highly pathogenic viruses and can be maintained in the agricultural sector with minimal or no involvement of wild birds. Transmission is promoted in poultry flocks due to the practice of keeping them in densely packed intensive poultry farm and consequent close contact with secretions through which the virus can be transmitted. Highly pathogenic avian influenza viruses (including H5N1) can cause great mortality in domestic poultry flocks but have rarely been isolated from wild birds until recently. There is no known natural reservoir for highly pathogenic avian influenza viruses. They emerge normally after low pathogenic viruses jump from water birds into poultry. Samples collected from clinically normal birds in the wild have not yielded any H5N1 viruses, though epidemiological studies suggest that wild birds are likely to have played a role in the transmission of H5N1 viruses to domestic poultry. Interestingly, no one has uncovered the lineage of the H5N1 variant circulating in waterfowl in Southern China before the first known outbreak of the disease in chickens in Hong Kong in 1997. There is no evidence that H5N1 infections in humans have been acquired from wild birds. Human infections have occurred in people who have been closely associated with poultry. Wild waterfowl, especially ducks are natural reservoirs of avian influenza virus and may be an important source of infection in domestic waterfowl and poultry and provides a reservoirs of all H subtypes except H13. Wild birds may come into contact with farmed poultry directly or indirectly (via contaminated feed and water). The latter route is especially important for farmed duck reared on ponds and for poultry whose drinking water is obtained from ponds. Influenza viruses target the GI tract of waterfowl and ducks which can shed virus for as long as 10-30 days. As one of the wild bird's symptoms is diarrhea it could mean that virus would spread in contaminated water. The virus can persist and retain infectivity in water (>30 days at 0°C and up to 4 days at 22°C). The virus is transmitted through aerosol route if birds are in close proximity or direct contact with contaminated respiratory secretions or faecal secretions. Once introduced into a flock, the virus is spread from flock to flock by the usual methods involving the movement of infected birds and movement of contaminated fomites. Poultry birds can catch the infection through contact with wild birds and waterfowls. There is considerable body of circumstantial evidence to support the hypothesis that migratory waterfowl, sea birds or shore birds are generally responsible for introducing the virus into poultry. Virus may readily be isolated in large quantities from the faeces and respiratory secretions of infected birds. It is logical to assume that because virus is present in body secretions, transmission of the disease can take place through shared and contaminated drinking water. Birds are readily infected when there is instillation of virus into the conjunctival sac, nares or the trachea. Preliminary field and laboratory evidence indicates that virus can be recovered from the yolk sac and albumin of eggs laid by hens at the height of the disease. The possibility of vertical transmission is unresolved. However, it is unlikely that infected embryo could survive and hatch. The disease is highly contagious and one gram of contaminated manure can contain enough HPAI virus to infect 1 million birds.

12

Low Pathogenicity Avian Influenza (LPAI) and High Pathogenicity Avian Influenza (HPAI): Symptoms and Lesions

Clinical Signs

The pathotype of AI virus (LP or HP) has a major impact on the clinical manifestation of the disease. However, clinical signs of the disease are extremely variable and depend on host species, age, sex, concurrent infections, acquired immunity and environmental factors.

Low Pathogenic AI Viruses

Most infections by LPAI viruses in wild birds produce

no clinical signs. However, in domestic poultry (chicken and turkeys), clinical signs are coughing, sneezing, rales, rattles and excessive lacrimation. Abnormalities in the digestive, urinary and reproductive symptoms are also noticed. In layers and breeder, hens may exhibit increased broodiness and decreased egg production. Besides, huddling, ruffled feathers, depression, decreased activity and decreased water and feed consumption and occasionally diarrhea has been reported. Emaciation is less frequently reported.

Highly Pathogenic Avian Influenza (HPAI) Viruses

In wild birds and domestic ducks, HPAI viruses replicate poorly and produce few clinical signs. In domestic chickens, turkeys and related galliformes, damage to multiple visceral organs, cardiovascular and nervous systems is noticed. The disease is fulminating in some chickens or turkey in a flock causing death prior to the observation of any clinical signs. If the disease is less fulminating, birds survive for 3-7 days, exhibiting nervous disorders such as tremors of head and neck, inability to stand, torticollis and opisthotonus. Depression is common due to less feed and water consumption. Precipitous drop in egg production occur in breeders and layers. Respiratory symptoms include rales, sneezing and coughing.

In ostriches (*Struthio camelus*), reduced activity and appetite, depression, ruffled feathers, sneezing and open mouth breathing have been reported. Some birds show incoordination, paralysis of wings and tremors of the head and neck.

Morbidity and Mortality

In chickens, turkeys and related *Galliformes* birds, morbidity and mortality rates are as variable as the signs and are dependent on virus pathogenicity and the host as well as age, environment and concurrent infections. For the LPAI, high morbidity and low mortality rates (<5 per cent) is typical unless accompanied by secondary bacterial infections. With the HPAI viruses, morbidity and mortality rates are very high and can reach up to 100 per cent in some flocks.

In wild birds, LPAI viruses usually produce no mortality or morbidity. In ostriches, LP and HP avian influenza viruses usually produce moderate morbidity and low mortality. But mortality rates as high as 80 per cent have been reported for LP avian influenza viruses in chicks less than one month of age.

Gross Pathology

The appearance of gross lesions is variable depending on the virus strain, the length of time from infection to death and the age and species of poultry affected. Clinical signs, lesions and death have been seen with domestic poultry of the Order *Galliformes*, Family *Phasianidae* but not of the Order *Anseriformes* or *Charadriiformes* when infected with HPAI viruses.

HPAI Viruses

In poultry, HPAI produce a variety of oedematous, haemorrhagic and necrotic lesions in visceral organs and the skin. In peracute cases, death occurs without showing any gross lesions. In chickens, swelling of head, face, upper neck and feet are common due to subcutaneous oedema and accompanied with petechial haemorrhages. Necrotic foci, haemorrhages and cyanosis of the non-feathered skin is common especially wattles and combs. Haemorrhages on serosal or mucosal surfaces of the visceral organs particularly epicardium, pectoral muscles and proventriculus are noticed. Necrotic foci are common in pancreas, spleen, heart, liver and kidney. The lungs can be congested or haemorrhagic with diffuse interstitial pneumonia accompanied with oedema. The cloacal bursa and thymus are usually atrophic. The pancreas may have red to light orange to brown mottling. Ruptured ova with 'yolk peritonitis' have been reported in layers and broilers and turkey breeders.

LPAI Viruses

LPAI in poultry birds may produce lesions in respiratory tract especially the sinusitis and tracheitis with thickened mucous and catarrhal, fibrinous and mucopurulent inflammation. The tracheal mucosa can be oedematous with congestion and haemorrhages. Microscopically there is diffused pneumonia, heterophilic to lymphocytic tracheitis and bronchitis, nephrosis and nephritis, pancreatitis, lymphocyte depletion and apoptosis of lymphocytes in the bursa, thymus and spleen.

Histopathology

Histologic lesions are most consistent in tissues having gross lesions and depends on the virus strain, inoculum, breed of chicken and route of inoculation. In general, the histologic lesions consist of multi-organ necrosis, and/or inflammation. Brain, heart, lung, pancreas, primary and secondary lymphoid organs are severely affected.

The HPAI virus causes sudden deaths of birds in peracute cases but necrosis and inflammation is generally lacking in parenchymal cells of most visceral organs, brain and skin. If present, such lesions are mild and multifocal in distribution. Most consistently the HPAI virus replicates in the vascular endothelial cells and cardiac myocytes causing generalized cell death.

In acute cases, the prominent lesions are necrosis and less commonly inflammation, haemorrhages, oedema and apoptotic cell death. If the bird survive for longer time, the more prominent the inflammation and less prominent the necrosis or apoptosis.

Lesions are found in most of the visceral organs, most prominently in the brain, heart, pancreas, kidney, adrenal and skin. Lymphocytic meningoencephalitis with focal gliosis, neuronal necrosis and neuronophagia are common but oedema and haemorrhage may be seen. Focal degeneration to multifocal diffuse coagulative necrosis of cardiac myocytes has been reported accompanied with lymphohistiocytic inflammation. Necrosis in skeletal muscle, kidney tubules, vascular endothelial cells, corticotrophic cells of adrenal and pancreatic acinar cells is less commonly observed. In lymphoid tissue, necrosis, apoptosis and depletion are common in cloacal bursa, thymus and spleen.

The non-feathered skin contains numerous microthrombi within dermal and hypodermal capillaries and small blood vessels. It is accompanied by vasculitis, generalized oedema, subcutaneous oedema and necrosis of capillary endothelium.

13

Transmission of Influenza Virus between Species

Influenza viruses are usually species specific. That means swine influenza virus circulates only among pigs, equine influenza virus among equines, avian influenza virus among birds and human influenza viruses among humans. Occasionally, these viruses cross species barriers. Generally the virus is not well adapted to the new host and does not undergo sustained transmission.

Transmission of avian influenza virus to people is rare and has been reported only with H5, H7 and H9 viruses. Most infections have been the result of direct contact with infected poultry or fomites. No cases of person to person transmission with the avian viruses have been noticed to date.

The H5N1 avian influenza virus may be likely to undergo cross species transmission. These viruses have been isolated at least 56 times in humans after contact with infected poultry. But rarely transmission between species results in an epidemic in the new host. Generally this requires a novel H and/or N protein to evade the immune response together with viral proteins that are well adapted to the new host cells. Occasionally, a virus is transferred whole to the new host and can spread. However, dissemination is more likely if the novel virus reassorts with a virus that is already adapted to the new host. Reassortment can occur in the new host's own cells. It could also occur in an intermediate host particularly pigs. Pigs have receptors that can bind swine, human and avian influenza viruses. For this reason, they have been called mixing vessels for the formation of new viruses.

Although reassortment can occur anywhere in the world but many of the new viruses originated in Asia. In rural China and other regions, a variety of species including ducks are kept in close proximity to each other and to humans facilitating the increased opportunity for virus reassortment.

The last three human pandemic appear to have been the result of the reassortments. The 1957 H2N2 (Asian flu) virus contained avian H, N and an internal protein (PB1) and 5 other proteins from human H1N1 strain. The H3N2 Hong Kong flu virus of 1968 had two new protein from an avian virus [the new H and an internal protein (PB1)] but N and other proteins from the H2N2 virus. The origin of the strain that caused the 1918 human pandemic (Spanish flu) is uncertain. Although the haemagglutinin protein is more closely related to avian influenza virus than to human influenza virus, there is some evidence that this virus may have evolved in an intermediate host before causing an epidemic in humans. Repeated reassortments of human, avian and swine influenza virus have also resulted in novel swine viruses.

Reassortant HPAI viruses may become progressively more virulent for mammals. From 1999 to 2002, H5N1, avian influenza virus isolated from healthy ducks in Southern China acquitted the ability to replicate and cause lethal disease in mice. Most of the viruses appear to be reassortants that contain a H gene related to A/Goose/Guangdong/1/96 (H5N1) HPAI virus and other genes from unknown Eurasian avian influenza virus.

14

Criteria for Classifying the Avian Influenza Viruses into HPAI and LPAI

Out of the two glycoproteins (H and N) present on the surface of the AI viruses, H appears to be the most important protein in determining the virulence of AI viruses. The virulence of the virus has no link with the type of N protein present along with the H protein. Many disease conditions caused by LPAI viruses may even appear sometimes as mimicking the symptoms of HPAI but there are certain criteria which must be fulfilled before declaring the AI virus infection as HPAI.

To date the presence of multiple basic amino acids (arginine and lysine) motifs at their HA cleavage sites has been demonstrated only for a limited number of field isolates of AI virus belonging to H5 or H7 subtypes. These viruses have been assigned to the HPAI viruses, in order to distinguish them from all other virus strains which are responsible for low pathogenicity avian influenza (LPAI). The LPAI H5 viruses have basic amino acid at position–1 and–4 and LPAI H7 viruses at –1 and –3 of HA cleavage site whereas multiple basic amino acids are present in H5 and H7 HPAI viruses.

H5 subtypes of low virulence have amino acid sequence at HA0 cleavage site.

PQRETR*GLF

PQKETR*GLF

H5 subtypes of high virulence have amino acid sequence at HA0 cleavage site.

PQRKRKTR*GLF

PQRKKR*GLF

PQRETRRRQKR*GLF

PQKKKR*GLF

PQRKRKTR*GLF

PQRERRRKKR*GLF

PQRERRRKKR*GLF

PQRRRKKR*GLF

H7 subtypes of low virulence have amino acid sequence at HA0 cleavage site.

PEIPKGR*GLF

PENPKGR*GLF

H7 subtypes of high virulence have amino acid sequence at HA0 cleavage site.

PEIPKKKKR*GLF

PETPKRKRKR*GLF

PEIPKKREKR*GLF

PETPKRRRR*GLF

R = arginine K = lysine

OIE Protocols

1. Any influenza virus that is lethal for 6 or more of eight 4-8 weeks old susceptible chickens within 10 days following I/V inoculation of 0.2 ml of a 1/10 dilution of bacteria free infective allantoic fluid.
2. The following additional test is required if the isolate kills 1 to 5 chickens but is not of H5 or H7 subtypes: growth of the virus in cell culture (for example primary cells such as chick embryo cells or cell lines such as MDCK cells, although most cell cultures support the growth of HPAI and LPAI viruses in the presence of trypsin) with CPE or plaque formation in the absence of trypsin. If no growth is observed the isolate is not considered to be a HPAI isolate.
3. For all H5 and H7 viruses of low pathogenicity and for other influenza viruses, if growth is observed in cell culture without trypsin, the amino acid sequences of H must be determined. If the sequence is similar to that observed for other HPAI isolates, the isolate is considered as highly pathogenic.

All the HPAI strains isolated to date have possessed either the H5 or H7. Further information concerning the pathogenicity of H5 or H7 subtypes may be obtained by sequencing the genome as pathogenicity is associated with the presence of multiple basic amino acid (arginine or lysine) at the cleavage site of HA0. However, two isolates (H10N4 and H10N5) killed 7/10 and 8/10 chickens with intravenous pathogenicity index (IVPI) values >1.2 when the birds were inoculated intravenously. But they produce no death signs when inoculated intranasally and these did not have multiple basic amino acids at the H cleavage site.

EU Protocols

Pathogenicity Test

An infection of poultry caused by an influenza A virus is considered highly pathogenic if the I/V pathogenicity index in 6 weeks old chicken is >1.2 or any infection with influenza A viruses of H5 or H7 subtype revealed the presence of multiple basic amino acid at the cleavage site of HA0.

Intravenous Pathogenicity Index (IVPI)

1. Fresh infective fluid with a HA titre >1/16 is diluted 1/10 in sterile saline solution.
2. 0.1 ml of diluted virus is injected I/V into ten 6 weeks old SPF chickens.
3. Birds are examined at 24 hours intervals for 10 days. At each observation, each bird is scored 0 if normal, 1 if sick, 2 if severely sick and 3 if dead.
4. The IVPI is the mean score per bird per observation over the 10 day period. An index of 3.0 means that all the birds died within 24 hours and an index of 0 means that no birds showed any clinical signs during the 10 days observation period.

15

Influenza Pandemics

An influenza pandemic is defined as a global outbreak of disease that occurs when a new strain of influenza A virus emerges in the human population causing serious illness and then spreads easily from person to person worldwide. Pandemic viruses mainly originated from antigenic shift and major changes caused by new combinations of the H and N proteins on the surface of the virus. Most of the pandemics have originated in parts of Asia where dense populations of human live in close proximity to ducks and pigs. The temporary banning of public gatherings and closure of schools may be effective measures to help delay the international spread of a pandemic. The true influenza pandemics are unmistakable and may have catastrophic consequences. The twentieth century witnessed 4 pandemics all of which spread throughout the world within a year of being detected.

First Pandemic

It is called Spanish flu (H1N1) which occurred between 1918 and 1919 and caused highest number of known deaths, more than 0.5 million in the USA and possibly as many as 50 million worldwide. Most of the deaths occurred within a few days of the person being infected, and nearly half of those who died were young healthy adults. The H1N1 was reintroduced into the human population in the 1970s. Phylogenetic and sero-archeological studies suggest that all genes of the 1918 pandemic strain were closely related to those of H1N1 swine viruses. Phylogenetic analysis of sequences encoding the H, N, NP, M1 and M2 proteins disclosed a genetic relationship between the pandemic strain and H1N1 human and swine influenza A viruses. Further study of the H gene indicated the absence of multiple basic amino acid at the cleavage site in contrast to findings in virulent avian viruses.

Second and Third Pandemics

The second pandemic is called Asian Flu (H2N2) occurred 40 years later (1957-1958) and caused 70,000 death in the USA. It was identified first in China in February, 1957 and reached the USA by June of that year. The third pandemic occurred a decade later in 1968-1969, called Hong Kong flu (H3N2). The disease was detected in Hong Kong in early 1968 and later that year reached the United States causing death of 34,000 humans. The human pandemic viruses, such as those responsible for Asian influenza (H2N2) in 1957 and Hong Kong influenza in 1968, share two important features: they first emerged in southeastern Asia and they were antigenically distinct from the influenza viruses then circulating in humans. Genetic studies, together with biochemical analyses indicated that Asian and Hong Kong pandemic strains were generated by reassortment between human and avian viral genes. The causative virus in the 1957 pandemic possessed 3 genes [PB1, H (H2) and N(N2)] from an avian virus and all remaining genes from a circulating human H1N1 virus which disappeared soon after the H2N2 virus emerged. The pandemic H3N2 virus identified in Hong Kong in 1968 was a reassortant with avian PB1 and H (H3) genes and six other genes from a human H2N2 virus. It is suggested that antigenic shift occurred as result of reassortment of genes in dual infections with viruses of human and avian origin. The H2N2 influenza virus could no longer be detected in humans after the H3N2 influenza virus appeared. Phylogenetic studies indicated that the avian viral genes in these pandemic strains were derived from viruses of Eurasian lineage, originated in Southern China. Although many people died during these pandemics, the causative viruses do not seem to be extraordinarily pathogenic unlike 1918 strain. The increase in death rate associated with these viruses was probably as a result of the lack of immunity to these viruses in human populations. It is noteworthy that both Asian and Hong Kong outbreaks were caused by hybrid viruses or reassortants that harboured a combination of avian and human viral genes. Avian influenza viruses are therefore key contributors to the emergence of human influenza pandemics.

Fourth Pandemic

It is called Russian flu. The causative agent (H1N1) of the pandemic in 1977 was essentially identical to viruses circulating among humans in the 1950s. The relatively low death rate in this pandemic can be attributed to the immunity of persons over 20 years of age who had been infected with the virus when it circulated earlier in the country.

Sl.No.	*Year*	*Name of the Pandemic*	*Subtype of Influenza Virus*	*Death*
1.	1918-19	Spanish Flu	H1N1	50 million
2.	1957-58	Asian Flu	H2N2	70,000
3.	1968	Hong Kong Flu	H3N2	34,000
4.	1977	Russian Flu	H1N1	Relatively less

Most of the influenza pandemics in humans was due to reassortant viruses originated after undergoing the process of antigenic shift. Highly pathogenic avian influenza viruses are constant threat to poultry industry only until the Hong Kong outbreak (H5N1), there was no zoonotic evidence that avian viruses could be transmitted directly to humans. The identification of avian viruses in humans to cause devastating influenza outbreaks in major human populations pose a potential pandemic threat. In March 1999 in Hong Kong, an H9N2 avian influenza virus was isolated from two children with mild influenza symptoms. Genetic studies showed that all the genes other than the H and N were closely related to those of the H5N1 viruses, suggesting the role of these genes in efficient transmission of the virus from birds to humans. In fact, surveillance of live poultry markets in Hong Kong in December, 1997 revealed the presence of H9N2 viruses in addition to H5N1 viruses in birds in these markets. It is speculated that future influenza pandemics will probably be caused by an avian virus possessing an H surface protein to which humans lacks immunity. Whether this virus will be introduced directly or indirectly into human populations is uncertain, but at least two mechanisms seem plausible. So, when entire human population of the world is at risk to an influenza pandemic outbreak, scientist, researchers and academicians should have to be vigil and alerted to tackle/ overcome that situation to avert any outbreaks by some means in the form of immunoprophylactic or therapeutic agents.

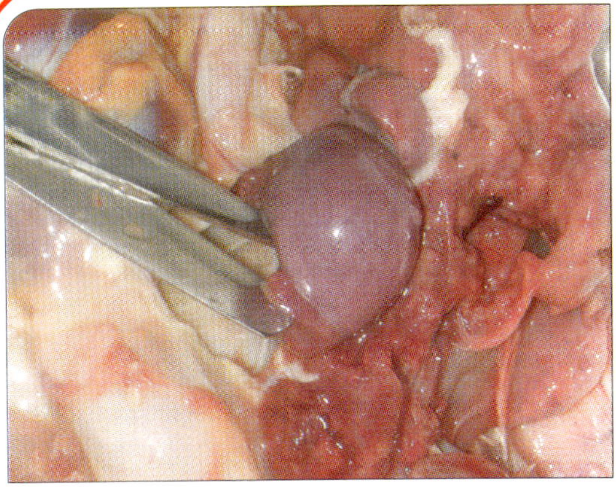

Congestion and Harmorrhages of Spleen of a Avian Influenza Affected Bird

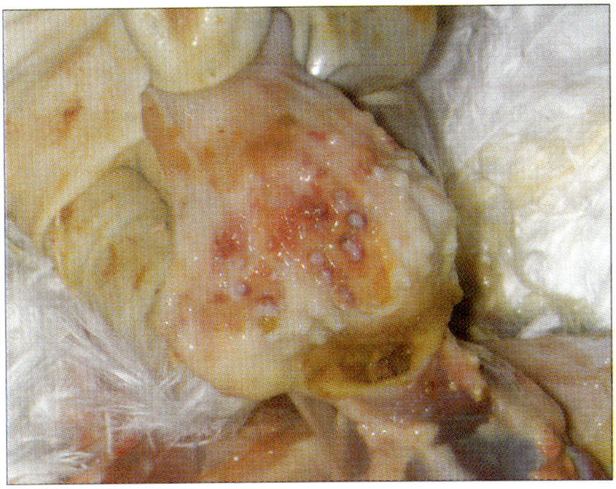

Haemorrhages in the Proventiculus

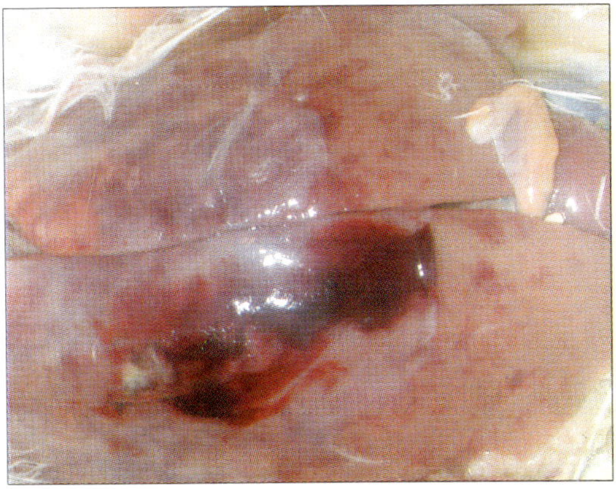

Haemorrhages of the Liver of a Bird Flu Affected Bird

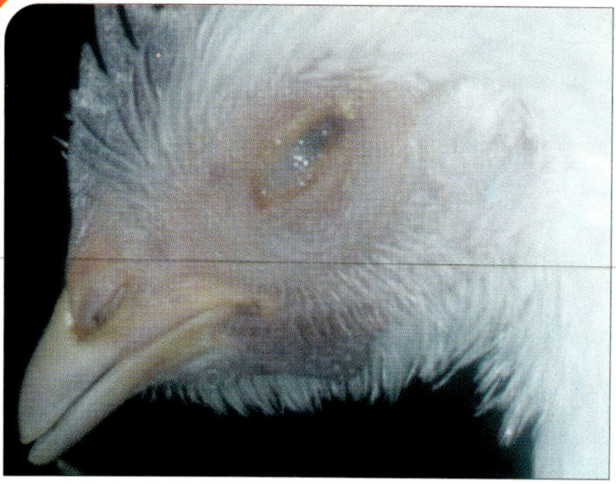

Ocular Discharge from a Avian Influenza Affected Bird

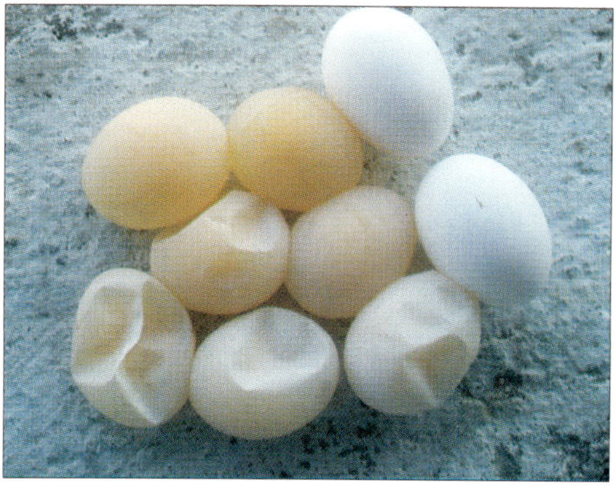

Production of Soft Shelled or Misshaped Eggs from Avian Influenza Affected Bird

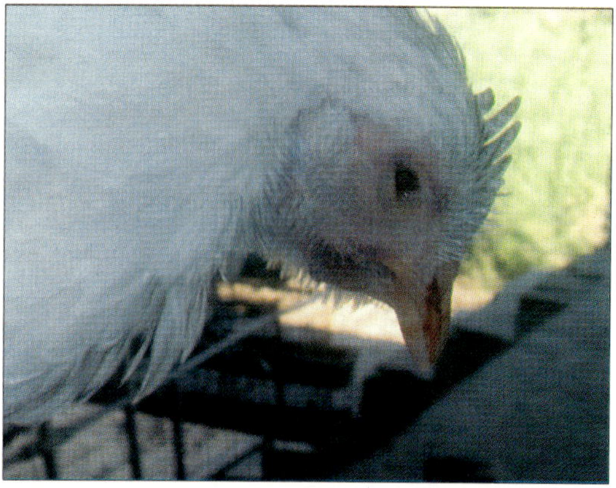

Bloody Discharge from Mouth and Purplish Discoloration of the Wattle

16

Recent Major Outbreaks of Avian Influenza

Historically avian influenza viruses have been extremely rare findings in humans. They caused only mild illness, usually viral conjunctivitis, followed by a full recovery. Influenza viruses arising from these avian hosts intermittently transmit to other avian and even mammalian species. However, viral replication in the aberrant host is usually limited and does not typically result in overt disease. Influenza outbreak in humans (H5N1) in Hong Kong in 1997 has proved to be an exception when an avian influenza virus was directly transmitted to the humans causing severe illness with high mortality. Pandemics are as unpredictable as the viruses that cause them and demonstrate great variations in mortality, severity of illness and patterns of spread. A rapid surge in the number of cases and their exponential increase over a brief period of time often in a matter of weeks, is a constant characteristic. The ability of the virus to cause severe disease in young adults is a major determinant of a pandemic's overall impact. The epidemiological potential of a virus tends to occur in waves with age groups and geographic areas initially not affected being likely to prove vulnerable during the next wave. It was suggested that pigs acted as 'mixing vessel' in which reassortment between human and avian influenza viruses could take place with the emergence of viruses with the necessary gene(s) from the virus of human origin to allow replicating and spread in the human population, but with a different H surface glycoprotein so that human population could be regarded as immunologically naïve. H5N1 is of particular concern because it mutates rapidly and has a propensity to acquire genes from viruses infecting other animal species. Its ability to cause severe disease and death in humans has been documented. The increasing incidence of H5N1 in birds and accompanying increase in opportunities for direct infection of humans pose the likelihood that humans concurrently infected with human and avian influenza strains could become "mixing vessels" for the emergence of a novel subtype with sufficient human genes to be transmitted easily from person to person.

17

Characteristics of Pandemic Influenza Viruses and Characteristics of 1997 H5N1 Hong Kong Influenza Virus

Characteristics of Influenza A Virus having Potential to Cause Eandemics

(*a*) They mutate much more rapidly than influenza B viruses giving them great flexibility.

(*b*) In addition to humans they infect pigs, horses, sea mammals and birds.

(*c*) They have numerous subtypes all of which are maintained in aquatic birds which provide a perpetual source of viruses and a huge pool of genetic diversity.

(*d*) They regularly cause seasonal epidemic in humans, with heavy tolls in mortality and morbidity.

(*e*) They undergo antigenic shift which serves well as a long term survival tactic.

Characteristics of the Influenza A H5N1 Virus (Hong Kong, 1997)

(*a*) It has become progressively more pathogenic in poultry and in the mammalian mouse model.

(*b*) The virus is HPAI for chickens and turkeys. Viral antigen was demonstrated in multiple tissues, confirming the pantropic nature of this avian species. However, there was a particular predilection for chicken/HK virus to localize in the vascular epithelium, heart, pancreas, brain and adrenal glands of the gallinaceous birds.

(*c*) The chicken/HK virus demonstrated only a modest ability to replicate in ducks, sparrows and gulls. Furthermore, pigeons, starlings, rats and rabbits were largely resistant to infection with H5N1 virus. In the ducks and gulls, the chickens/HK virus was primarily pneumotropic, causing only minimal to mild lesions within respiratory tissues.

(*d*) It is now hardier than previously and it survives several days longer in the environment.

(*e*) It appears to be expanding its mammalian host range.

(*f*) It has been found in its highly pathogenic form in dead migratory birds and the role of migratory waterfowl in the evolution and maintenance of highly pathogenic H5N1 may be changing.

(*g*) It has been found in its highly pathogenic form in domestic ducks which can excrete large quantities of lethal virus without warning signs of visible lesions.

(*h*) It is occurring in concentrated poultry outbreaks in rural areas, where most households maintain free ranging flocks and ducks and chickens mingle freely.

Recently symptomatic domestic ducks have been shown experimentally to excrete H5N1 in its highly pathogenic form. This finding poses a great concern because it indicates that ducks may play an important silent role in maintaining transmission. The ducks can excrete large quantities of lethal virus without showing warning signs of visible disease. The world's first cases of human infection with the avian H5N1 strain were documented in 1997 in Hong Kong. For the first time, evidence showed that the avian H5N1 strain can infect human directly without prior adaptation in a mammalian host. A striking feature of this outbreak was the presence of primary viral pneumonia in severe cases. Usually pneumonia that occurs in patients with influenza is a secondary bacterial infection. In these cases, however, pneumonia was caused directly by the virus, it did not respond to antibiotics and it frequently was rapidly fatal. The outbreak which involved 18 cases, six of which were fatal coincided with outbreaks of infection of H5N1 in domestic poultry farms and live markets. Within 3 days, the entire poultry population of Hong Kong was culled to avert a possible pandemic influenza outbreak in humans.

Further Incidence

The incidence of zoonotic avian influenza (H5N1) was reported again in 2003 that is currently persisting too, causing more human fatalities in few of the Asian countries since an outbreak in Hong Kong in 1997. Up to 12th March, 2008, 231 death out of 373 (62 per cent) human cases have been reported around the world from 37 countries. The countries where most of the human cases reported are Thailand, Vietnam, Indonesia and China. Apart from H5, it is also seen that H7 and H9 avian influenza virus has raised concern by trying to establish themselves among the human populations. Studies have indicated that H7N3, H7N7 and H9N2 subtypes are capable of jumping to humans, getting opportunities to swap genetic material with human strain which could result in a reassortant virus. Genetic, molecular and biological studies have shown that human infections could be possible with H5N1, H9N2, H7N7 and H7N3 subtypes of avian influenza viruses and all these subtypes have been isolated from human beings. However, H5N1 is of great concern at present as most of human casualties in recent years were due to this subtype of AI virus (H5N1).

18

Human Health Implications

Due to the recent cases of human infection caused by AI viruses and to the concern about the generation of a new pandemic virus originating from H5N1 virus, AI infections are now considered a significant threat for public health.

Although it has been known for sometime that the human pandemic viruses of 1957 and 1968 appeared to arise by reassortment between human influenza viruses infecting birds and AI viruses infecting humans, it was suggested that pigs which both human and avian viruses are known to infect readily acted as "mixing vessels". Reassortment between human and AI viruses could therefore take place in pigs, with the emergence of viruses with the necessary gene(s) from the virus of human origin to allow replication and spread in the human populations, but with a haemagglutinin surface glycoprotein of avian species, so that the human populations could be regarded as immunologically naïve.

The biggest threat resulting from the direct natural infections of humans with AI viruses is that pandemic viruses could emerge as a result without an intermediate host. There are two mechanisms by which this could occur: by genetic reassortment or by progressive adaptation. In the first mechanism, a hybrid or reassortant virus is generated when a person is simultaneously infected with an AI virus and a human influenza virus. This has been reported with virus containing H5, H7 or H9 haemagglutinin and having the potential for causing true influenza pandemic.

The second mechanism by which the generation of a pandemic virus may occur is through progressive adaptation of a virus entirely of avian origin. Recent studies on the genome of the H1N1 'Spanish influenza' virus have speculated that the virus was entirely of avian origin and not generated by reassortment. The virus harboured all the eight segments of avian origin and killed more persons than World War I.

Regardless of the mechanism by which the new human pandemic virus may be generated, it appears logical that AI virus circulation should be reduced or avoided. This is one of the most complex problems in developing countries. The human cases that have occurred during the ongoing H5N1 epidemic have developed following contacts between villagers and rural chickens/fighting cocks. The nature and entity of these contacts are dependent on social and behavioural practices linked to food security or hobby activities. The basic hygienic standards are rarely respected. Efforts should be concentrated on the reduction of viral shedding from rural poultry so that the amount of virus shed is insufficient to infect a human beings. It is considered by many that vaccination interventions of rural poultry currently appear to be the only means to achieve a reduction of virus load in the rural environment. Lastly, bio-security encompassing bioexclusion and bio-containment of high standard and stamping out policy must be implemented and maintained to represent a firewall against the penetration and perpetuation of AI virus and minimize the infections of humans to a great extent.

Transmission

The disease is transmitted to humans by direct or indirect contact with infected aerosols and discharges as large quantity of viruses are excreted in birds through droppings and can survive for short time in the environment. There is no evidence of human to human transmission till date. So far no cases of human to human transmission by small particle aerosols has been reported. The risk of nosocomial transmission to health care workers has been low even when appropriate isolation measure were not followed. However, one case of severe illness was reported in a nurse exposed to an infected patient in Vietnam. Oral ingestion of contaminated water during swimming and direct intranasal or conjunctival inoculation during exposure to water and contamination of hands from infected fomites and subsequent infection are other potential modes of transmission. The widespread use of untreated poultry faeces as fertilizer is another possible risk factor.

Incubation Period in Humans

The incubation period of avian influenza (H5N1) may be longer than other known influenzas. The incubation period is 2-4 days but may extend up to 8 days.

Symptoms

Most patients have initial symptoms of high fever (>38°C) and influenza like illness with lower respiratory tract symptoms. Upper respiratory tract symptoms are present only occasionally. Unlike patients with infections caused by avian influenza A (H7) viruses, patients with avian influenza A (H5N1) rarely have conjunctivitis. Diarrhea, vomiting, myalgia, abdominal pain, pleuritic pain and bleeding from the nose and gums have also been reported early in the course of illness in some patients. Watery diarrhea without blood and inflammatory changes appears to be more common in H5N1 infections in humans with human influenza viruses and may precede respiratory manifestations. Two patients with encephalopathic illness and diarrhea without apparent respiratory symptoms have also been available.

Clinical Course

Lower respiratory tract manifestations develop early in the course of illness. Dyspnoea developed usually 5 days after the onset of illness. Respiratory distress and tachypnea are common. Sputum production is variable and sometimes bloody in nature. Most of the patients have pneumonia, radiographic changes include diffuse, multifocal and interstitial infiltrates with segmental or lobular consolidation. Usually primary viral pneumonia is evident without bacterial superinfection.

The respiratory failure may be associated with diffuse, bilateral infiltrates with acute respiratory distress syndrome manifestations. Multi-organ failure with signs of renal dysfunction including cardiac dilatation and supraventricular tachyarrhythmias has been common. Other complications included ventilator associated pneumonia, pulmonary haemorrhages, pneumothorax, Reye's syndrome and sepsis without bacteremia.

Mortality

The fatality rate among the hospitalized patients has been high although the overall rate is probably much lower. In 1997 most of the death occurred among patients older than 13 years of age whereas recent avian influenza A (H5N1) causes high rates of death in infants and young children. The case fatality rate was 89 per cent in patients younger than 15 years of age in Thailand. Death usually occurs due to respiratory failure in 9-10 days after the onset of illness.

Laboratory Findings

Leukopenia, particularly lymphopenia, mild to moderate thrombocytopenia, slight to moderate increase of aminotransferase levels are commonly observed. Marked hyperglycemia may be due to the use of cortisone. The level of creatinine is also increased. In Thailand, an increased risk of death was associated with decreased leukocyte, platelet particularly lymphocyte counts.

Diagnosis

The presumptive diagnosis is made based on the history and clinical symptoms. A patients is suspected for avian influenza (bird flu) if he or she has any respiratory illness and has had recent direct or indirect contact with sick chickens or other birds. The X-ray of the chest may be useful in detecting early viral pneumonia. Nasopharyngeal aspirate, endotracheal aspirate, sputum and serum from clinically suspected cases are collected for further laboratory examination to provide the confirmatory diagnosis.

The diagnosis of influenza A (H5N1) can be confirmed by virus isolation in Hep-2, RD cells or MDCK cell lines followed by identification in immunofluorescence assay/ ELISA using specific monoclonal antibodies (MAbs). Unlike human influenza A infection, avian influenza A (H5N1) infection may be associated with a higher frequency of virus detection and higher viral RNA levels in pharyngeal than in nasal samples. Detection of influenza specific RNA by reverse-transcriptase–Polymerase chain reaction (RT-PCR) using primer sets specific for H5 and N1 can provide the sensitive, specific and accurate result. Serological identification by measuring the specific antibodies by HI, ELISA and virus neutralization test (VNT) more specifically micro-neutralization test have also been developed.

Rapid antigen assays may help to provide a diagnosis of influenza A infection but they have poor negative predictive value and lack specificity for influenza A (H5N1). Laboratory confirmation of influenza A (H5N1) requires one or more of the following: a positive viral culture, a positive RT-PCR assay for influenza A (H5N1) RNA, a positive immunofluorescence test for antigen with the use of monoclonal antibodies against H5 and at least 4 fold rise in H5 specific antibody titer in paired serum samples.

Pathological Lesions

Severe pulmonary injury with histological changes of

diffuse alveolar damage has been reported both in human influenza with H5N1 virus infection and other human influenza A viruses. Alveolar space with fibrinous exudates and RBC, vascular congestion, infiltration of lymphocytes into the interstitial areas and proliferation of reactive fibroblasts are noticed. Antemortem biopsy of bone marrow specimens has shown reactive histiocytosis with hemophagocytosis; whereas lymphoid depletion and atypical lymphocytes have been observed in spleen and lymphoid tissues at autopsy. Centrilobular hepatic necrosis and acute tubular necrosis have also been noted in several cases.

19

Treatment of Bird Flu Infections in Humans/ Anti-viral Agents

If bird flu is suspected in a person, treatment should be started immediately without waiting for laboratory confirmation. Four antiviral drugs (Amantadine, Rimantadine, Zanamivir and Oseltamivir) have been approved by the US Food and Drug Administration (FDA) for treatment of influenza. The drugs need to be taken within 2 days after becoming sick. The drugs can reduce flu symptoms and may shorten the time of sickness by 1 or 2 days and make the patients less contagious. All these drugs must be taken under medical supervision and are 70-90 per cent effective in preventing illness in healthy adults. All the above anti-viral drugs may be effective against influenza A viruses but Oseltamivir and Zanamivir are effective for influenza B viruses also. Oseltamivir and Zanamivir block the function of the viral neuraminidase. In 1997, human cases of influenza A (H5N1) infections were treated with Amantadine in Hong Kong. This anti-influenza drug prevents viral infection by interfering with M-2 ion channel activity, thus inhibiting virus uncoating. It provided complete protection in chickens against viral infection. Withdrawal of the drug and rechallenge with the lethal virus results in death of all chickens. A single mutation confers resistance to the drug against both human and avian influenza viruses. Virus infected chickens treated with Amantadine survived but shed drug resistant viruses that were lethal to contact birds. Hence, Amantadine offers prophylaxis against influenza virus infection but is not ideal for treatment of active disease. Again, the current strain of H5N1 has already shown resistance to Amantadine and Rimantadine, two anti-viral drugs commonly used for influenza.

Other drugs namely Oseltamivir and Zanamivir are still effective against influenza viruses by inhibiting the neuraminidase enzyme. These viruses are susceptible in vitro to these drugs. One of drugs Zanamivir (Relenza, Glaxo Welcome Inc) is inhaled as a powder twice a day for 5 days. A special device called a disk inhaler is supplied with the medication. The other drug, Oseltamivir phosphate (Tamiflu TM, Roche Pharmaceuticals) is available in the form of tablet that is taken orally for 5 days.

Oral Oseltamivir and topical Zanamivir are active in animal models of influenza A (H5N1). Recent murine studies indicate that as compared with an influenza A (H5N1) strain from 1997, the strain isolated in 2004 requires higher

Oseltamivir doses and more prolonged administration (8 days) to induce similar anti-viral effects and survival rates.

Early treatment will provide the greatest clinical benefits, although the use of therapy is reasonable when there is a likelihood of ongoing viral replication. Approved doses of Oseltamivir (75 mg in adults or weighing more that 40 Kg, 60 mg for 23-40 Kg, 45 mg for 15-23 Kg and 30 mg for 15 kg or less for 5 days twice daily) are effective in treating early, mild cases of influenza A (H5N1). None of the anti-virals are approved for use in children under 1 year of age. Higher doses of 150 mg twice daily can be used in adults for 7 to 10 days. Oseltamivir is marketed as trade name Tamiflu by Roche and Zanamivir as trade name Relenza by Glaxo Wellcome Inc.

High level anti-viral resistance to Oseltamivir has been reported in influenza A (H5N1) virus due to substitution of a single amino acid in N1 neuraminidase (His274Tyr). Such variants have been detected in up to 16 per cent children with human influenza (H1N1) who have received Oseltamivir. The resistant variant has also been detected recently in patients with influenza A (H5N1) who were treated with Oseltamivir. The new variants are less infectious in cell culture and in animals compared to susceptible parental virus. However, such variants retain full susceptibility to Zanamivir and partial susceptibility to the new neuraminidase inhibitor (under investigation) Peramivir in vitro. Besides Zanamivir and Peramivir, other drugs of choice are long acting neuraminidase inhibitor Ribavirin and possibly IFN-α.

Tamiflu is not a stomach irritant and can be taken with or without food. But if Tamiflu is taken with food, the lesser are the chances of stomach upsets. Tamiflu should be taken for a minimum of 5 days and its should not be abruptly ceased if the patients begins to feel better.

Taking Tamiflu may have some side effects depending on the patient to patient. The side effects of Tamiflu may range from mild to severe and includes cough, phlegm production, wheezing, nausea, vomiting, diarrhea, stomach cramps, stomach upsets, nose bleed, itching of eyes, redness of eyes, headache, insomnia and dizziness. In case the side effects become intolerable, discontinue use of Tamiflu and consult doctor for further action.

20

Avian Influenza and Human Death

According to WHO, in the year 2003, there were 4 cases of avian influenza in humans with 100 per cent mortality (China-1 and Vietnam–3). In 2004, 17 cases were reported from Thailand only with death of 12 people. In 2005, five countries namely Cambodia (4 death out of 4), Indonesia (13 out of 20), Thailand (2 out of 5), China (5 out of 8) and Vietnam (20 out of 61) reported the avian influenza in human beings. The highest number of deaths in human beings due to avian influenza were reported in the year 2006 which include 9 countries [Azerbaijan (5/8), Cambodia (2/2), China (8/13), Djibouti (0/1), Egypt (10/18), Indonesia (45/55), Iraq (2/3), Thailand (3/3) and Turkey (4/12)]. In the year 2007, 59 deaths out of 86 cases of avian influenza in humans has been reported from China

(3/5), Egypt (9/25), Indonesia (37/42), Lao People's Democratic Republic (2/2), Pakistan (1/1), Vietnam (5/8) and Nigeria (1/1). So, a total of 236 people died due to bird flu out of 373 people affected from 2003 to 18th March, 2008. The details has been given in the table.

Country	*Death/ Cases (Year)*	*Total Deaths*
China	1/1 (2003), 5/8 (2005), 8/13 (2006), 3/5(2007), 3/3 (2008)	20
Vietnam	3/3 (2003), 20/29 (2004), 19/61 (2005), 5/8 (2007), 5/5 (2008)	52
Thailand	12/17 (2004), 2/5 (2005), 3/3 (2006)	17
Cambodia	4/4 (2005), 2/2 (2006), 1/1 (2007)	7
Indonesia	13/20 (2005), 45/55 (2006), 37/42 (2007), 10/12 (2008)	105
Azerbaijan	5/8 (2006)	5
Djibouti	0/1 (2006)	0
Egypt	10/18 (2006), 9/25 (2007), 1/4 (2008)	20
Iraq	2/3 (2006)	2
Lao People's Democratic Republic	2/2 (2007)	2
Nigeria	1/1 (2007)	1
Turkey	4/12 (2006)	4
Pakistan	1/1 (2007)	1
Maynmar	0/1 (2007)	0
Total	236/373	236

From the table, it is evident that highest number of human casualties has been reported from Indonesia (63) followed by Vietnam (42), Thailand (17), China (14) and Egypt. In Djibouti, only one case was reported without any human casualties.

21

Collection of Samples and Diagnosis of Avian Influenza

Collection of Sample

Both the tracheal and cloacal swabs, although swabs of the latter site are more suitable to yield the virus, should be collected from live birds. The collection of fresh faeces may serve as an adequate alternative. Oro-nasal swabs, cloacal swabs and intestinal contents (faeces) are collected from dead birds. Samples of trachea, lungs, air sacs, intestine, spleen, kidney, brain, liver and heart may also be collected and processed either separately or as a pool.

The samples should be placed in PBS, pH 7.0-7.4 containing antibiotics (Penicillin 2000 units/ml, Streptomycin–2 mg/ml, Gentamycin 50 µg/ml and

Mycostatin–1000 units/ml) for tissues and tracheal swabs but at 5 fold higher concentration for faeces and cloacal swabs and sent to the laboratory on ice.

Processing of Sample

Faeces and finely minced tissues are prepared as 10-20 per cent suspension in PBS containing antibiotics followed by centrifugation at 1000 g for 15 minutes. Supernatant is collected and kept at –20°C until further use.

Inoculation into Eggs

The supernatant fluid is inoculated into the allantoic sac of at least 5 SPF hen eggs of 9-11 days old. The eggs are incubated at 35-37°C for 4-7 days. Eggs containing dead or dying embryos are chilled at 4°C and allantoic fluid should then be tested for HA activity.

Diagnosis

(*a*) AGID

All the influenza A viruses have antigenically similar nucleocapsid and matrix protein. Concentrated virus preparation contain both matrix and nucleocapsid antigens. The matrix protein antigen diffuse more rapidly than nucleocapsid antigen in the AGID test. AGID has been widely and routinely used to detect specific antibodies in chicken and turkey flocks as an indication of infection. The infected chorioallantoic membrane (CAM) of embryonated hen's egg is homogenized freeze-thawed three times and centrifuged at 1000 g for 15 minutes. The supernatant fluids are inactivated by the addition of 0.1 per cent formalin or 1 per cent BPL, recentrifuged and used as antigen in the AGID test. However, not all avian species may produce precipitating antibodies following infection with influenza viruses. For subtyping the virus, the laboratory must have monospecific antiserum prepared against the isolated antigens of each of the different H and N proteins.

(*b*) Haemagglutination Test

It can be used to diagnose the avian influenza virus infections. It is carried out by adding 25 ul of two fold dilution of antigens in PBS in V shaped microtitre plate followed by addition of 25 ul of PBS and 25 ul of chicken RBC (1 per cent) to each well. The plate is incubated at room temperature for 40 minutes or 60 minutes at 4°C. Suitable controls are also included in the test. The titre is expressed as the highest dilution of antigen given complete HA which is designated as 1 HA unit.

(*c*) Haemagglutination Inhibition Test

It can be used to know the specificity of the avian influenza virus as demonstrated by the inhibition of the haemagglutination of chicken RBC in the presence of antiserum raised against avian influenza virus. It is carried out by adding 25 ul of 2 fold dilution of antiserum made in PBS in the V shaped microtitre plate followed by addition of 25 ul of antigen containing 4 HA units to all the wells. 25 ul of chicken RBC is added to all the wells and plate is incubated at 40 minutes at room temperature or 60 minutes at 4°C. Suitable controls are also included in the test. The HI titre is the highest dilution of serum causing complete inhibition of 4 HA units of antigens.

Reverse Transcriptase–Polymerase Chain Reaction (RT-PCR)

It serves as a fast and effective alternative to virus isolation for the detection of influenza viruses. The subtype specific primers are used to amplify the part that flank the sequence encoding for cleavage site of HA protein (HA1+HA2). This is an important tool to discriminate the HPAI viruses from LPAI viruses as they differ in bearing the multiple basic amino acid sequence at the cleavage site of HA protein.

Nucleic Acid Hybridization

In this method parts of NP, M and HA genes of H5, H7 and H9 of avian influenza virus are amplified, cloned into plasmid vectors and can be used as hot and cold DNA probes to screen large number of influenza A viruses.

22

Prevention, Control and Eradication

In emergency disease outbreaks, large number of poultry may need to be killed for control, containment and eradication purposes. Live poultry present the major risk of spreading infectious agents so their slaughter must be completed humanely and as quickly as possible. Various strategies have been adopted for prevention, control and eradication of avian influenza throughout the world. Actions vary from no action on some LPAI viruses to the extreme of stamping out or depopulation programmes for eradication of HPAI. Individual countries have chosen control and eradication programmes to meet the domestic expectation. Measures taken to prevent, control or eradicate avian influenza will depend on the pathogenicity of avian influenza viruses, types of birds infected, geographic distribution of infected birds, requirement of domestic and international markets and economic status of the nation. With regards to HPAI, prevention should be limited to strategies to preclude introduction and exposure of poultry to the virus. However, if HPAI does occur, eradication is the only viable option. On the other hand, control implies reduction in incidence to a low or economically manageable level. A control programme is acceptable strategy for some strains of LPAI but not an acceptable option for an OIE list A disease such as HPAI. For control and eradication programme the following measures to be taken:

(1) Comprehensive, integrated national surveillance and diagnostic programme to know the disease status in a country.

(2) Enhanced biosecurity practiced at all the level of production and processing by all employees of companies, diagnostic laboratory and government agencies that have contact with poultry or equipments.

(3) Education of poultry farmers and other workers about avian influenza control and sharing of information on surveillance and control strategies at all the levels in the production process.

(4) Quarantine and controlled movement of avian influenza infected poultry.

(5) Vaccine can be used as comprehensive control programme under government control.

(1) Surveillance and Diagnostics

A comprehensive, integrated surveillance and diagnostic programme is essential to determine the magnitude of avian influenza virus infections in commercial and live bird market, domestic poultry and migratory and non-migratory wild birds. Such information is essential to establish the national or regional prevalence of LPAI and HPAI within a country and affect the import and export potential of poultry and poultry products and other related avian commodities. A national or regional veterinary medical diagnostic facility is essential to make rapid and accurate diagnosis of avian and to characterize the virus isolates as LP or HP. The rapid diagnosis of HPAI cases is essential as it will allow to rapidly eliminate the disease before additional birds are infected and disease becomes endemic.

(2) Biosecurity

Enhanced biosecurity, an important part of any avian prevention and control serves two purposes.

(*a*) Containment of the avian influenza virus on infected farms (biocontainment)

(*b*) prevention of introduction the virus to the naïve farms (bioexclusion).

The practice of biosecurity must be implemented at all the levels within the poultry industry and allied groups and by all employes involved. It includes proper disinfection and decontamination of all equipment used on more than one farm, precautions to avoid carrying of virus in faecal and respiratory secretions in boots, clothing and shoes and involvement of workers restricted to one farm operations.

(3) Educations

Education and dissemination of information to poultry farmers and other workers, veterinarians, Govt. officials and media about the avian influenza and biosecurity measures to be practiced for the successful prevention and control of the programme.

23

Methods for Killing Poultry in the Event of an Avian Influenza Outbreaks

Inhalation Agents

CO_2, CO, N_2, argon, HCN, Halothane, methoxy fluorane and isofluorane.

Injectable Anaesthetics

Injectable anaesthetics can be also be used.

Physical Method

Electrocution, cervical dislocation, decapitation and maceration.

Recommendations of WHO on AI

Avian influenza is a highly contagious disease of birds

which is currently epidemic amongst poultry in Asia. Exposure to infected poultry and their faeces or dust/soil contaminated with faeces can result in human infection. In view of any outbreak the following measures are to be followed.

1. Cullers and transporters should be provided with protective clothing covers alls plus an impermeable apron, heavy duty rubber gloves and N95 respirator masks. Goggles, rubber or polyurethane boots that can be disinfected or protective foot covers that can be discarded.
2. Persons who are in close contact with infected birds should wash their hands frequently with soap and water. Cullers and transporter should disinfect their hands after operation.
3. All the persons exposed to virus suspected for avian influenza should be under close monitoring by local health authorities.
4. It is recommended that Oseltamivir (Tamiflu–Roche) or Zanamivir (Relenza–GSK) be readily available for the treatment of suspected H5N1 respiratory infection in culler and farm workers involved in mass culling. They should be vaccinated with the current WHO recommended vaccine to avoid simultaneous infection by human influenza and avian influenza and to minimize the possibility of a reassortment.

24

Avian Influenza in Wild Birds

Although domestic chickens and turkeys are susceptible to severe and potentially fatal influenza A caused by highly pathogenic avian influenza (HPAI) virus strains, it can infect a variety of the domestic and the wild avian species (including chickens, turkeys, ducks, domestic geese, quails, pheasants, patridge, psittacines, gulls, seabirds, shorebirds, emu, eagles and others). The clinical manifestation of infection in birds ranges from asymptomatic infection to rapidly fatal diseases. Aquatic birds particularly Anseriformes (ducks and shorebirds) and Charadriiformes (gulls and terns) are considered as naturals reservoirs for avian influenza viruses. These waterfowls generally donot develop disease when infected with avian influenza viruses, however, H5N1 appears to be virulent for a variety of wild bird species. Domestic ducks are susceptible to influenza A virus infections and virus replicate in the cell lining of the intestinal tracts without producing any clinical signs but shedding the virus up to 5 days post infection. An outbreak of H5N1 among migratory geese and other wild birds in Quinghai province, China was identified in May, 2005. An outbreak in wild swans occurred in Azerbaijan in February, 2006 and severe illness from H5N1 influenza recently has been recognized in a variety of other wild birds species. Recent studies showed that North Americans wood ducks and laughing gulls are susceptible to illness and death from HPAI H5N1. Investigators in Asia showed that asymptomatically infected domestic ducks shed more H5N1 influenza virus for longer periods in 2004 than in 2003, which may be a factor in amplify the spread of H5N1 to domestic poultry. Another report demonstrated the presence of H5N1 influenza virus in asymptomatic eagles that were smuggled from Thailand into Belgium in 2004. HPAI H5N1 viruses were isolated from asymptomatic tree sparrows in the Henan province of China in 2005.

Influenza A viruses have traditionally been known to cause disease in horses, pigs whales and seals, however, the range of several influenza A subtypes is expanding to different mammalian species. H5N1 influenza A has now been shown to infect cats, leopards, tigers, civets and dogs. H5N1 recently was isolated from an infected mink and a stone marten in Europe. A recent report involving cats experimentally infected with H5N1 demonstrated that infected cats excreted the virus via the respiratory tract and the digestive tract suggesting that in addition to the respiratory route, other routes of transmission may play a role in spread among mammalian hosts. Cat to cat transmission of H5N1 can occur. H5N1 was also identified in pigs in China in 2001 and 2003.

25

Avian Influenza in Tigers and Leopards

Influenza A viruses have been isolated from a variety of animals, including pigs, horses, minks, seals, whales, birds and humans. Interspecies transmission of influenza viruses although rare, has been detected. Although influenza viruses can infect a wide variety of birds and mammals, the natural hosts of the virus is wild waterfowl, shorebirds, and gulls. When other species of animals, including chickens, turkeys, swine, horses and humans are infected with influenza viruses, they are considered aberrant hosts. Influenza viruses undergo a high rate of antigenic mutation called antigenic shift. The evolutionary rate of influenza virus in the natural host reservoirs is slow, while in mammals the rate is much higher. Due to the mutation, many different viral genotypes will co-circulate in the host, with each virus potentially having different levels of fitness for the environment. The advantage of a high error rate is the ability of viruses to rapidly adapt to a new environment. This is required during infection of a new host species that required favourable genetic changes for optimal replication and transmission. The disadvantage of the high error rate is the production of many viral genotypes that are defective or have reduced fitness for the current host.

The high degree of nucleotide and amino acid sequence homology of the genes coding for the internal proteins suggests that influenza viruses are well adapted to their natural hosts. Well adapted viruses will cause only subclinical or mild disease, but they will replicate and shed in sufficient concentration to allow efficient transmission to other susceptible hosts. For examples, avian influenza virus in migratory ducks is well adapted without causing any disease. However, when influenza virus crosses into a new host species in which it is not adapted, the virus can cause severe disease.

Although viruses with all H and N are found in avian species, viral subtypes of mammalian influenza viruses are limited. Those which have circulated widely in humans are restricted to 3 H and 2 N (H1, H2 and H3: N1 and N2 subtypes). During the H5N1 virus outbreak in Thailand in December, 2003, two tigers (*Panthera tigris*) and two leopards (*P. pardus*) at a zoo in Suphanburi, Thailand showed clinical signs, including high fever and respiratory distress and died. The animals had been fed fresh chicken carcasses from a local slaughter house. At that time many chickens around Suphanburi were dying with respiratory symptoms due to avian influenza (H5N1) virus infection.

Post-mortem Findings

The primary gross lesions in all the four animals were severe pulmonary consolidation and multifocal haemorrhages in lung, heart, thymus, stomach, liver, lymph nodes and intestine. Histological findings revealed that loss of bronchiolar and alveolar epithelium, thickening of alveolar walls and lumen filled with edema fluid mixed with fibrin, RBC, neutrophils and macrophages.

Confirmatory Diagnosis

The disease was further confirmed by reverse-transcriptase polymerase chain reaction (RT-PCR) using the primer pairs specific for the H and N genes and found positive for avian influenza H5N1. Sequencing and phylogenetic analysis of the H and N genes of virus isolated from the tigers and leopards showed that they were virtually identical to each other and to the H5N1 virus circulating in poultry at that time. Therefore it is concluded that the tigers and leopards were most probably directly infected with avian influenza A (H5N1) virus by feeding on infected poultry carcasses. Lung samples from all four animals negative for canine distemper virus by RT-PCR and one which is positive for a vaccine strain of feline panleukopenia virus administered 2 weeks before death.

Influenza A virus can also cause death in non-domestic felids. Generally, influenza virus is also not considered pathogenic for the domestic cat. Experimental infection of domestic cats in the 1970s and 1980s with influenza A viruses of subtypes H3N2 from humans and H7N3 from a turkey and H7N7 from a harbour seal *(Phoc vitulina)* resulted in transient virus excretion and a temporary increase in body temperature but did not induce clinical signs of the disease. However, anecdotes of fatal infection have been reported in this species during the 2003-2004 H5N1 virus outbreak.

From this finding, it is clear that influenza A viruses can infect tigers and leopards besides domestic cats and H5N1 virus is more pathogenic for felids than other influenza viruses. This findings has important implications for wild life conservation and epidemiology of influenza viruses. It may also be included in the list of the emerging viruses affecting the wildlife. The influenza H5N1 virus infection may threaten the survival of endangered wildlife *viz.*, tigers and leopards and the severity of the threat is increased because H5N1 virus may be transmitted horizontally between felids. Again, the higher pathogenicity of H5N1 virus for felids means excretion of more virus over a long period of time. So, the role of felids in avian influenza epidemiology both in humans and in poultry needs to be again reevaluated. Finally, the death of leopard and tigers, two other mammalians besides humans implied that more species of mammals needs to be screened because they may be at risk for infection with this virus.

26

Laboratories Authorized to Test Samples Suspected for Avian Influenza

The avian influenza or bird flu, a highly contagious and infectious disease of birds has become a major concern due to devastating consequences on the poultry industry and having the zoonotic potential to cause the disease in humans. However, there are other disease conditions which may show the signs and symptoms similar to bird flu. Avian influenza can also be divided into LPAI and HPAI (bird flu) based on the clinical manifestation and mortality patterns. So, the diagnosis of the disease should be carried out promptly, precisely and accurately so that unnecessary panicking can be avoided. The virus isolate can be characterized from High security Animal Disease laboratory, Bhopal or abroad. However, the detection of LPAI of H5 and H7 subtypes is a matter of concern as it may mutate to give rise to the HPAI virus. The list of the laboratory given in the article will be of extreme help in diagnosing the disease conditions in poultry and necessary measures can be taken to tackle the situation efficiently.

In India:

Dr S.C. Dubey

Joint Director cum Station Incharge
High Security Animal Disease Laboratory,
Anand Nagar, Bhopal–462 021, M.P.
Ph: 0755-2759204 (O), 0755-2754683 (R)
Mobile: 09425606992
Fax: 0755-2758842, E-mail: scd2009@yahoo.co.in

Abroad

List of OIE Reference Laboratories and Other Experts for Highly Pathogenic Avian Influenza

Dr Ortrud Werner

National Reference Laboratory for Highly Pathogenic Avian Influenza and Newcastle Disease,
Institute of Diagnostic Virology, Federal Research Centre for Virus Disease of Animals (BFAV)
Insel Riems, Boddenblick 5a, 17493 Greifswald–Insel Riems
GERMANY/ ALLEMANGE/ALEMANA
Tel: (41) 383.517.152 Fax: (41) 383.517.151
E-mail: ortrud.werner@rie.bfav.de

Dr Ian Brown

VLA Weybridge
New Haw, Addlestone, Surrey KT15 3NB

UNITED KINGDOM/ROYAUME/REINO UNIDO
Tel: (44.1932) 34.11.11 Fax: (44.1932)34.70.46
E-mail: i.h.brown@via.defra.gsi.gov.uk

Dr Paul W. Selleck

CSIRO, Australian Animal Health Laboratory (AAHL)
5 Portarlington Road, Private Bag 24, Geelong 3220, Victoria
AUSTRALIA
Tel: (61.3)52.27.50.00 Fax: (61.3)52.27.55.55
E-mail: paul.selleck@csiro.au

Dr B. Panigrahy

National Veterinary Services Laboratories
P.O. Box 844, Ames, IA 500 10
USA/EE.UU
Tel: (1.515) 663.75.51 Fax: (1.515) 663.73.48
E-mail: brundaban.panigrahy@aphis.usda.gov

Dr Ilaria Capua

Instituto Zooprofilattico Sperimentale delle Venezie,
Laboratorio Virologia
Via Romea 14/A 35020 Legnaro, Padova
ITALY
Tel: (39.049)808.43.69 Fax: (39.049)808.43.60
E-mail: icapua@izsvenezie.it

Dr H. Kida

Graduate School of Veterinary Medicine,
Hokkaido University, Department of Disease Control
Kita-18, Nishi-9, Kita-ku, Sapporo 060-0818
JAPAN/JAPON/JAPON

Tel: (81.11) 706.52.07 Fax: (81.11)706.52.73
E-mail: kida@vetmed.hokudai.ac.jp

Other Experts

Dr David Swayne
Southeast Poultry Research Laboratory
USDA/ARS
934 College Station Road
Athens, Georgia, USA
Tel: 001-706-546-3433 Fax: 001-706-546-3161
E-mail: dswayne@seprl.usda.gov

Dr Veronique Jestin
Unite de pathologie aviaire
Zoopole Beaucemaine-Les Croix
BP 53, 22440 Ploufragan
FRANCE
Tel: (033(0)2) 96.01.62.81
Fax: (033(0)2) 96.01.62.73
E-mail: v.jestin@ploufragan.afssa.fr

27

Vaccines Against Avian Influenza

Various strategies have been used for prevention, control and eradication of AI throughout the world. Strategies include no action on some LPAI viruses to the extreme of implementing stamping out or depopulation programme for eradication of HPAI. The use of vaccine to control AI has been widely debated. Although not officially prohibited, vaccination of poultry against LPAI infections other than those caused by H5/H7 viruses is only occasionally performed. Although there is a general agreement, for the need to discourage the use of specific vaccines, immunization of turkeys and chickens has been carried out against H5/H7 LPAI or HPAI. Individual countries have chosen control or eradication programme as per the domestic expectations. Measures taken to prevent control or eradicate AI will vary depending on the pathogenicity of the AI viruses, types of birds infected, geographical distribution of infected birds, requirement of domestic and internation markets and economic status of the nation. In case of HPAI, prevention should be limited to strategies to preclude introduction and exposure of poultry to the virus. However, if HPAI does occur, eradication by slaughtering the infected birds is the only viable option.

Vaccines

Vaccination is the most cost effective method available to prevent and control the avian influenza and to minimize the huge economic losses and increasing the lifespan of the birds against the particular disease. The vaccines against AI can be divided into 7 different types.

1. Inactivated homologous vaccine
2. Inactivated heterologous vaccine
3. Split vaccine
4. Live attenuated vaccine
5. Recombinant DNA vaccine
6. DNA vaccine
7. Transgenic plant vaccine

1. Inactivated Homologous Vaccine

Influenza virus vaccines were first developed in the 1940s and consisted of partially purified preparations of influenza viruses grown in the embryonated eggs. Due to the presence of egg derived components, these formaldehyde inactivated vaccines were highly pyrogenic and lacking in efficacy. In the 1960s, the use of ultracentrifuge revolutionized the purification process and better vaccines with improved safety, potency and efficacy could be produced. Inactivated homologous vaccine is prepared from the prevalent strain of AI virus grown in the embryonated egg inoculated through allantoic route. The allantoic fluid is collected, inactivated with either formaldehyde or BPL and used as vaccine to control the HPAI. The vaccine is found to be highly efficacious and used in Mexico and Pakistan. The disadvantage of this vaccine is that the vaccinated birds cannot be differentiated from the infected ones.

2. Inactivated Heterologous Vaccine

The vaccine is prepared in the same way as in above. But the strain of AI virus used in the vaccine is of same H type but has a different or heterologous N type. The advantage of the vaccine is that antibody against N protein can be used as marker and vaccinated birds can be differentiated from the infected birds. It has been used against H7N1 (field strain) in Italy in 2002 by incorporating H7N3 strain of AI virus in the vaccine preparation. The vaccine is licensed to use in many countries. Aventis Pasteus Global prepared the inactivated vaccine based on this technology for use in the human beings and trial is currently being undertaken.

3. Split Vaccine

Most influenza virus vaccines used in the US and Europe consists of embryonated egg grown and formaldehyde inactivated preparations which after purification are disrupted with a non-toxic detergent (Triton X-100). The split virus preparations show lower pyrogenicity than whole virus vaccines. In general, 1 dose for adult contains 45 μg HA (15 μg HA for each of the 3 antigenic components, an H1N1 influenza A, an H3N2 influenza A and an influenza B). This dose is approximately the amount of purified virus obtained from the allantoic fluid of 1 infected embryonated egg. If 100 million doses of killed influenza virus vaccine are to be prepared, the manufactures has to procure 100 million embryonated eggs. The manufacturer of the vaccine is clearly dependent on the timely availability of embryonated eggs and the vaccine strains to be used in a particular season. Most of these prototype seed strains are provided to the manufacturers by Government agenies which create high yielding strains through classical reassortment with a high yielding laboratory strains A/PR/8/34. Unfortunately only high yielding influenza A viruses can be made in this way and 6:2 reassortants (HA and NA from recently circulating strains and remaining 6 genes from A/PR/8/34 virus) are sometimes not easily obtained. Subsequently, in 2005–2006, vaccine formulation is made up of the A/New Caledonia/ 20/99 (H1N1), A/California/7/2004 (H3N2) and B/ Shanghai/361/2002 viruses. Changes in the HA of circulating viruses (antigenic drift) require periodic replacement of the vaccine strains with the current field strains. This process of reassortment is time consuming and followed by repeated passage of the strain in embryonated eggs to allow for egg adaptation and growth enhancement. Influenza B virus prototype strain with good growth characteristics are usually obtained by direct and repeated passaging in embryonated eggs without attempting to generate reassortants. Although the manufacturing process is time consuming, these killed influenza A and B virus vaccines are the workhorses for vaccination against influenza and have been shown to be highly effective from time to time.

4. Live Virus Vaccines

The only FDA licensed product against influenza is the cold adapted attenuated vaccine. In this process, influenza virus was passaged at 25°C in chicken kidney cells and embryonated eggs. It is a clod adapted, temperature sensitive and highly attenuated master strain. The annually updated vaccine strains are generated in the laboratory by reassortment with viruses more closely related to the currently circulating ones. The resulting vaccine strains (both A and B types) are 6:2 reassortants with 6 internal proteins genes derived from the cold adapted master strains and the HA and NA from circulating A and B viruses, reflecting the changing antigenicity.

Advantages

1. The vaccines can be easily administered by nasal spray.
2. They induce both local mucosal neutraling immunity and cell mediated responses.
3. The duration of immune response is longer and more cross reactive than those elicited by inactivated vaccine preparation.
4. No need to add any adjuvants.
5. Vaccine efficacy in vaccine naïve children 6 months to 18 years of age is high (range 73-96 per cent) and increased to 82-100 per cent after second shot.

Despite the obvious efficacy of both killed and live influenza virus vaccines, there is room for further developments. Among the critical issues in developing new and better vaccine are (1) price per dose (2) speed of production (3) ease of production (4) choice of substrates to grow the virus or to express the viral antigens (5) cross protection for variant strains (6) efficacy in general and in immunologically naïve populations (7) safety and (8) acceptance by the regulatory agencies and the public.

5. Recombinant DNA Vaccines

Current FDA licenced influenza vaccines are based on the technologies developed in 1960s or earlier as described before. With the breakthrough of reverse genetics techniques, infectious influenza viruses from plasmid DNAs transfected into tissue culture cells can now be produced/ rescued. This technology permits the construction of the high yield 6:2 seed viruses by mixing the 6 plasmid DNAs cloned with 6 internal protein genes from a good growing laboratory strain with the HA and NA DNAs of a currently circulating strain. It takes only 1-2 weeks period, to generate seed viruses for distribution to the manufacturers. The backbone of the 6:2 recombinant viruses could be prepared, tested and distributed in advance. Similar approaches can be adopted for the manufacturing of live, cold adapted influenza virus vaccines. In this case, the backbone would consist of the 6 genes of the cold adapted master strain and HA and NA from the currently circulating strains and produced employing reverse genetics system. Such an approach would have several advantages over the present manufacturing process.

1. It would dramatically accelerate the time frame for obtaining seed viruses for annual production and allow more time to select the appropriate seed strain.
2. It would standardize the seed viruses to be used.

3. The cloning of DNA coding for respective gene may eliminate the adventitious agents present in the throat washings of the original isolate.
4. Removal of the basic cleavage peptide by reverse genetics results in a virus that is attenuated for embryonated eggs and allowing high yields to be attained. The current highly pathogenic H5 strains (viruses that contain HA containing multibasic amino acids at HA1/HA2 cleavage site) kill embryonated eggs and personnel involved in manufacturing those vaccines.
5. Modification by reverse genetics results in a product that is easier to manufacture and safer to handle.

Live Influenza Virus Vaccine wither Altered NS1 Gene

The NS1 protein of influenza viruses has IFN antagonist activity. Influenza viruses that lack NS1 cannot counter the IFN response of the host. Thus infection of cells with virus of intermediate virulence and ability to induce IFN, one can construct ideal influenza virus that are both attenuated and highly immunogenic. IFN appears to be an excellent adjuvant that enhances production of immunoglobulin and contributes to the activation of dendritic cells required for antigen presentation. In this process, lower doses of live virus vaccine are required to induce a robust and protective immune response compared to conventional live or killed virus vaccines. If a 100 fold lower dose is required, many more people could have access to influenza virus vaccines. Moreover, live virus vaccine may give protective immunity in immunologically naïve populations after a single administration whereas killed virus vaccines may require high antigenic mass and booster doses. The live influenza virus vaccines appear to be more effective in immunologically naïve populations and a more economical way (intranasal) of vaccinating a large numbers of people.

Replication Defective Vaccines

In this process, influenza virus which lacks the gene for the nuclear export protein (NEP, formerly NS2) will go through a single cycle of replication without forming infection particles. Virus particles without M2 gene may also behave in this manner. The large scale production of defective viruses can be achieved by using complementing cell lines. The administration of virosomes (consisting of reconstituted viral envelopes that lack RNA) and the virus like particles made by expression of viral proteins have also been shown to be effective immunization strategies against influenza.

Vaccinia/Baculovirus Vector Influenza Vaccine

Vaccines produced with low and highly pathogenic H5 and H7 viruses had been prohibited in USA between the 1980 and 1995. A recombinant fowl pox vaccine containing HA or HA/NA of H5 and H7 ubtypes of AI virus is licensed to be used in Mexico, USA and El Salvador since 1998 against LPAI caused by H5N2 viruses. However, the protection afforded by recombinant fowl pox HA vaccines is reduced in chickens previously vaccinated against fowl pox or exposed to field strains of fowl pox virus. In experimental studies vaccinia virus or baculovirus expressed-HA vaccines have been shown to provide good protection against lethal infection by avian H5 and H7 subtypes.

Herpesvirus of Turkey Vector Influenza Vaccine

Although herpesvirus of turkey (HVT) had been indicated as a potential candidate for the development of an avian HA recombinant vaccine recently, vaccination of chickens with infectious laryngotracheitis virus recombinants expressing the HA gene of a H5 HPAI virus isolated in Italy in 1998, has provided protection from a lethal challenge with two distinct H5 HPAI viruses.

6. Nucleic Acid Vaccine

One of the first nucleic acid vaccines ever for use against AI was developed in 1993. The H7 gene was cloned into an expression plasmid containing the cytomegalovirus immediate early promoter and was shown to protect birds from a lethal challenge with AI virus of H7 subtype. The H7 DNA vaccine has been tested to have exerted protective immune response against homologous challenge with H7N1 AI virus. Plasmids encoding HA proteins of H7 and H5 subtypes have also shown to confer protection against HPAI viruses of both subtypes.

7. Transgenic Plant Vaccine

The expression of HA protein in transgenic plants has been recently indicated as a new strategy for immunization of poultry since oral vaccination with different live or inactivated preparations has been shown to confer protection against AI in chickens.

Vaccines Used in the Field

Vaccination has been proved to be a most cost effective way to prevent and control a disease. Historically, AI vaccines have been used mostly in the USA as part of a control programme against sporadic outbreaks of LPAI in meat turkeys. Between 1979 and 1997, a total of 22,385,000 doses of inactivated avian influenza vaccines were used, but generally vaccines against H5 and H7 subtypes have been discouraged by the USDA. A common use of vaccines has been to protect turkey breeders against sporadic outbreaks of moderately pathogenic swine H1N1 influenza viruses.

Although vaccines have been demonstrated to be protective against avian influenza, vaccination was not used in control and eradication programme against HPAI until 1995, in Mexico and Pakistan. However, in Mexico vaccines have continued to be used to control LPAI (H5N2) in broiler chickens, with 1.2 billion doses of inactivated AI vaccine and 0.3 billion doses of recombinant fowl pox vaccine with AI H5 gene insert used between 1995 and 1999. In general, vaccines should be used only if the number of HPAI cases is increasing and the disease is not contained within a single quarantine zone. Vaccine application should be limited to poultry within quarantine zones, ring vaccination around the periphery of the quarantine zone or vaccination to protect poultry pedigree stock within a region during an expanding HPAI outbreak.

Since the 1970s, inactivated vaccines have been extensively used in the USA against non-H5/H7 LPAI. In particular, a high number of doses of vaccines have been used in Minnesota from 1979 to 1997 to control outbreaks of LPAI in turkeys. H9N2 inactivated vaccines has been used to immunize turkeys against several outbreaks of AI in Germany. Inacitvated H6N2 and H9N2 whole virus vaccines are currently licensed to be used in Italy.

Summary

Since it is well known that although vaccination protects the birds from clinical signs and death, it does not prevent the virus circulation or mutation. In addition, it was possible that masking the clinical condition would lead to greater perpetuation of infection. Another point stressed the expert committee was that vaccination with an H7 vaccine would mask clinical signs caused by an HPAI virus that might arise by mutation. The movement of viraemic birds (to the abattoir) or to other establishments (young breeders) and movement of dead birds and infected litter, which were identified as being among the primary sources of infection should be totally stopped.

Arguments for the potential use of vaccines are mainly advocated on the basis of economic and social consequences of AI outbreaks. In the case of HPAI, the unpredictable appearance, the severity of the disease and the adoption of very restrictive measures can be generally regarded as self limiting factors to the spread of infection and finally to its eradication.

Finally the Italian experience with HPAI shows that it is extremely difficult to control this disease in densely populated areas, especially if infection with LPAI is already widespread in the area and therefore in order to avoid similar situations, prevention systems should be implemented. Besides, a structural change in the industrial system that must inevitably take place in order to reorganize production, circuits, veterinary surveillance, quarantine and controlled marketing are also essential to prevent sanitary emergencies. In addition, education of farmers and staff to the basic concepts of biosecurity is possibly the most critical point in the eradication of AI and fundamental to the management of poultry that are reared intensively.

For HPAI, an effective control or eradication programme has the following essential elements (1) Comprehensive integral national surveillance and diagnostic services (2) Enhanced biosecurity practiced at all levels of production and processing by all employees of companies, diagnostic laboratories and government agencies that have contact with poultry or equipment used for poultry operations (3) Quarantine of birds purchased/ imported and controlled movement of AI infected poultry and lastly (4) Use of vaccine as one element of a comprehensive control programme under national government control to tackle the most difficult situation.

28

Avian Influenza at a Glance

The bird flu has become a current, hot and burning topic now-a-days. The information about the disease has been given below to have knowledge about it at a glance and ready reference.

1. Avian influenza is caused by a virus under the genus *Influenzavirus A* and family *Orthomyxoviridae*. Other genera are *Influenzavirus B* and *Influenzavirus C* which do not affect birds.
2. Avian influenza viruses are enveloped and having 8 single stranded negative sense RNA as genome. They are very sensitive to most of detergents and disinfectants. Heating and drying readily inactivate them. However, viruses are well protected from inactivation by organic material and infectious

virus can be recovered in manure up to 105 days. Influenza viruses remain infectious 24 to 48 hours on non-porous environmental surfaces and 12 hours on porous surfaces outside the host. It can survive for 4 days in water at 22°C and 30 days at 0°C. The virus can be inactivated in 3 hours at 56°C and within 30 minutes at 60°C. Besides, acidic pH, SDS, lipid solvents, BPL, iodine compounds and formalin readily inactivate the virus. The virus is destroyed at 70°C within few minutes (a temperature much lower than the normal cooking temperature). So, consumption of properly cooked eggs and poultry meat is absolutely safe.

3. Influenza A viruses infecting poultry can be divided into two distinct groups on the basis of their ability to cause disease:low pathogenic avian influenza (LPAI) and highly pathogenic avian influenza (HPAI). The HPAI is a List A OIE disease and called bird flu but not the LPAI. LPAI is neither a list A nor a list B OIE disease.
4. The LPAI viruses usually cause subclinical or mild illness. The symptoms may include decreased egg production, mild to moderate respiratory disease and low mortality rate (5 per cent). More severe disease mimicking HPAI with high mortality rate of up to 50 per cent may also be seen in birds with LPAI when the condition is aggravated due to presence of secondary bacterial infection or other intercurrent viral diseases. The HPAI can cause serious disease in some species of birds on a farm while leaving others unaffected. The typical symptoms are oedema of head, cyanosis of the

head, comb and wattle, green to white diarrhea, blood tinged oral and nasal discharge, deformed or shell-less eggs production and neurological symptoms. Mortality may be as high as 100 per cent.

5. Influenza A viruses are also classified into subtypes based on the two surface antigens rod shaped haeagglutinin (H) and mushroom shaped neuraminidase (N). There are 16 different H and 9 different N antigens present in influenza A viruses. All the 16 H and 9 N in all the possible combinations (144 types) have been found in avian species whereas only limited viral subtypes have been observed in other species of animals.
6. In highly pathogenic avian influenza (HPAI) viruses, only H5 and H7 haemagglutinins have been found. HPAI viruses have intravenous pathogenicity index in 6 weeks old chickens >1.2, multiple basic amino acids (lysine of arginine) at the cleavage site of HA0 (precursor of H) and capability to grow and produce CPE or plaque in MDCK cells in the absence of trypsin.
7. The avian influenza viruses of subtype H5, H7 or H9 have been implicated to produce disease in humans and cause death in some cases.
8. Wild birds worldwide carry the influenza viruses in their intestines but usually do not get sick from them. However, domesticated birds, including chickens, ducks and turkeys can catch the infection when they come in contact with contaminated secretions or excretions and show the symptoms of the disease.

9. The antigenicity of avian influenza viruses change gradually by point mutations (antigenic drift) or drastically by genetic reassortment (antigenic shift). Both antigenic shift and drift have been observed in influenza A viruses but only drift in influenza B and C viruses.
10. The three pandemics of last century appear to have been the result of reassortments. The 1957 H2N2 (Asian flu) virus contained avian HA, NA and an internal protein (PB1) but 5 other proteins from a human H1N1 strains. The H3N2 Hong Kong flu of 1968 had HA and an internal protein (PB1) from avian species and remaining proteins from the H2N2 viruses. The origin of the strain that caused the 1918 human pandemic (Spanish flu) is uncertain but HA is more closely related to avian influenza viruses than human influenza viruses. There is some evidence that this virus may have evolved in an intermediate host before causing an epidemic in humans.
11. The influenza viruses are susceptible to a variety of disinfectants including 1 per cent Na hypochloride, 70 per cent ethanol, glutaraldehyde, formaldehyde and lipid solvent. It can also be inactivated at 56°C within 30 minutes, radiation and pH 2.0.
12. The diagnosis of influenza A (H5N1) can be confirmed by virus isolation in Hep-2, RD cells or MDCK cell lines followed by identification in immunofluorescence assay/ELISA using specific monoclonal antibodies. Besides, detection of influenza virus specific RNA by RT-PCR using

primer sets specific for H5 and N1 can provide the sensitive, specific and accurate result. Serological identification by measuring the specific antibodies by HI, ELISA and virus neutralization test (VNT) more specifically microneutralization tests have been developed.

13. The incubation period of avian influenza in humans is 2-4 days but may extend upto 8 days. Most patients show high temperatures (>38°C) and influenza like illness with lower respiratory tract symptoms. Fever, malaise, sore throat and cough are found in most of the patient while diarrhea, vomiting, abdominal pain, pleuritic pain and bleeding from nose and gums and conjunctivitis are seen in some patients. Persistent high fever is an useful signs. Life threatening complications like viral pneumonia, respiratory distress syndrome and multi-organ failure with signs of renal dysfunction including cardiac dilatation and supraventricular tachyarrhythmias may result in the death of the patients.
14. Aquatic birds such as ducks, shore birds and gulls are considered as natural reservoirs for avian influenza viruses. Generally, avian influenza virus infected waterfowl do not show the disease but carry and transmit the influenza viruses to other birds.
15. Influenza viruses are usually species specific. It means human influenza virus will infect human beings and avian influenza virus will infect birds. Avian influenza viruses bind to the sialyloligosaccharides terminated by sialic acid (SA)

α 2,3 galactose whereas human influenza viruses bind to the sialyloligosaccharides terminated by sialic acid (SA) α 2, 6 galactose. However, swine can be infected with swine influenza virus, human influenza virus and avian influenza virus because they have the receptors for both avian and human influenza viruses and considered as mixing vessels.

16. HPAI virus which is pathogenic for one avian species may not be pathogenic for another avian species. For example, ducks are typically resistant to viruses that are lethal to chickens.
17. The present understanding is that the HPAI virus has not been disseminated from wild birds to domestic poultry. However, H5 and H7 viruses are introduced to poultry flocks in their low pathogenic form and after circulating for few months they can mutate into the highly pathogenic form. The switching over from a low pathogenic avian influenza (LPAI) virus phenotype common in wild birds and poultry to HPAI virus phenotype is achieved by the introduction of basic amino acid resides into the HA0 cleavage site which facilitates virus replication.
18. The appearance of gross lesions is variable with HPAI virus infections and depends on the virus strain, length of time from infection to death and the age and species of bird affected. In general, clinical signs, lesions and death have been seen with domestic poultry of the order *Galliformes*, family *Phasianidae* but not in birds under *Anseriformes* or *Charadriiformes*.

19. Avian influenza viruses have been extremely rare finding in humans. They cause only mild illness usually viral conjunctivitis followed by a full recovery. In 1997, outbreaks of H5N1 in poultry in Hong Kong has been an exception as it transmitted from bird to human beings with 6 out of 18 people died.
20. The H5N1 is of particular concern as it mutates rapidly and has a propensity to acquire genes from viruses infecting other animal species including human beings. The infection of avian H5N1 virus in human concurrently infected with human influenza virus could emerge a novel subtype having the capability to be transmitted easily from person to person as human may act as mixing vessel.
21. The bird flu is transmitted to humans by direct or indirect contact with infected aerosols and discharges as large quantity of virus is excreted in birds through droppings. There is no evidence of human to human transmission till date. Oral ingestion of contaminated water during swimming and widespread use of untreated poultry faeces as fertilizer are other possible risk factors.
22. If bird flu is suspected in a person, treatment should be started immediately without waiting for laboratory confirmation. Four antiviral drugs (Amantadine, Rimantadine, Zanamivir and Oseltamivir) have been approved by the US FDA for treatment of influenza. The drug needs to be taken within 2 days after becoming sick. The drugs

can reduce flu symptoms and may shorten the time of sickness by 1 or 2 days and make the patients less contagious. All these drugs must be taken under medical supervision and are 70-90 per cent effective in preventing illness in healthy adults. All the above anti-viral drugs may be effective against influenza A viruses but Oseltamivir and Zanamivir are effective for influenza B viruses also. Oseltamivir and Zanamivir block the function of the viral neuraminidase. The current strain of H5N1 has already shown resistance to Amantadine and Rimantadine. However, Oseltamivir and Zanamivir are still effective against influenza viruses by inhibiting the neuraminidase enzyme. The viruses are susceptible *in vitro* to these drugs. The Zanamivir is marketed by Glaxo Welcome Inc as Relenza which is to be inhaled as powder for 5 days whereas Oseltamivir phosphate is marketed by Roche Pharmaceuticals as Tamiflu ™ which is to be taken orally as tablet for 5 days. Oral Oseltamivir and topical Zanamivir are active in animal models of influenza A (H5N1). Recent murine studies indicate that as compared with an influenza A (H5N1) strain from 1997, the strain isolated in 2004 requires higher Oseltamivir doses and more prolonged administration (8 days) to induce similar anti-viral effects and survival rates.

23. Early treatment will provide the greatest clinical benefits, although the use of therapy is reasonable when there is a likelihood of ongoing viral replication. Approved doses of Oseltamivir (75 mg in adults or weighing more that 40 Kgs, 60 mg for

23-40 Kgs, 45 mg for 15-23 Kgs and 30 mg for 15 Kg or less for 5 days twice daily) are effective in treating early, mild cases of influenza A (H5N1). None of the anti-virals are approved for use in children under 1 year of age. Higher doses of 150 mg twice daily can be used in adults for 7 to 10 days.

24. There are a number of OIE reference laboratories around the world, which work on avian influenza viruses and provide diagnosis. However, in India, only High Security Animal Disease Laboratory is authorized to test the samples suspected for avian influenza and provide diagnosis. For any enquiry, please write to:

Dr S. C. Dubey
Joint Director-cum-Station Incharge
High Security Animal Disease Laboratory,
Anand Nagar, Bhopal–462 021, M.P.
Ph: 0755-2759204 (O), 0755-2754683 (R)
Mobile: 09425606992
Fax: 0755-2758842, E-mail: scd2009@yahoo.co.in

Conclusion

Influenza remains an important disease of humans, animals and birds. It has become a burning topic when it was found that avian influenza virus can be directly transmitted to humans from poultry as it happened in 1997 in Hong Kong. Birds have been the primary source of zoonotic influenza A infections in humans in recent years in Asia. Transmission between humans is very limited at present but continued monitoring and surveillance is required to identify any increase in viral adaptation to human hosts. Avian influenza A (H5N1) in humans differs in multiple ways from influenza due to human viruses such as routes of transmission, clinical severity, pathogenesis and response to treatment. Unlike human influenza, avian influenza (H5N1) may have higher viral titers in the throat than in the nose hence analysis of throat swabs or lower respiratory samples may offer more sensitive means of diagnosis. Despite recent progress, knowledge of the epidemiology, natural history and management of influenza A (H5N1) disease in humans is incomplete. Recent human isolates of avian influenza A (H5N1) viruses are fully resistant of Amantadine and Rimantadine and few are resistant to Zanamivir also. So, bird flu having zoonotic potential has become a major concern and there is an urgent need to work on the area of the new drug discovery in order to obtain the more potent and effective drugs against human infections with avian influenza A (H5N1) viruses without any or minimal side effects which in turn safeguard the human life from the threat of the disease to a great extent.

Most of the influenza pandemics in humans were due to reassortant viruses originated after undergoing the process of antigenic shift. Highly pathogenic avian influenza viruses are constant threat to poultry industry only until the Hong Kong outbreak (H5N1) in 1997, there was no zoonotic evidence that avian viruses could be transmitted directly to humans. The identification of avian viruses in humans to cause devastating influenza outbreaks in major human populations pose a potential pandemic threat. Transmission between humans is very limited at present but continued monitoring and surveillance is required to identify any increase in viral adaptation to human hosts. It is speculated that future influenza pandemics will probably be caused by an avian virus possessing an H surface protein to which humans lacks immunity. Whether this virus will be introduced directly or indirectly into human populations is uncertain, but at least two mechanisms seem plausible–reassortment between the avian and human influenza viruses in the human beings or reassortment between these two viruses in the pigs acting as mixing vessels. With the appearance of H5N1 highly pathogenic avian influenza (HPAI) virus infections in human during 1997, it is possible that direct reassortment between AI and human influenza A viruses could occur within the human without the need for an intermediate host. As was the case in 1957 and 1968, an avian-human reassortant virus is the most likely candidate as the next pandemic strains. Humans as well as swine must now be considered a potential mixing vessel for the generation of such a virus. Efficient transmission among humans is a key property of pandemic strain. At present when entire human population of the world is at risk to a influenza pandemic outbreak, scientist, researchers and academicians should have to be vigilant to tackle/overcome that situation to avert any outbreaks by some means in the form of immunoprophylactic or therapeutic agents. So, bird flu having zoonotic potential has become a major concern and there is an urgent need to work on the area of the new drug discovery in order to obtain the more potent and effective drugs against human infections with avian influenza A (H5N1) viruses without any or minimal side effects which in turn safeguard the human life from the threat of the disease to a great extent. Newer technologies in the field of diagnosis, immunoprophylactic agents and anti-viral drugs would definitely emerge with the holistic approach and concerted efforts of people from all corners of the society to minimize the casualties of human beings from avian influenza or bird flu in foreseeable future.

References

Alexander, D.J. (2000a). A review of avian influenza in different poultry. *Vet. Microbiol.*, 74: 3–13.

Alexander, D.J. (2000b) The history of avian influenza in poultry. *World Poultry*, p. 7–8.

Banks, J., Speidel, E. and Alexander, D.J. (1998). Characterization of an avian influenza A virus isolated from a human is an intermediate host necessary for the emergence pandemic influenza viruses? *Arch. Virol.*, 143: 781–787.

Beare, A.S. and Webster, R.G. (1991). Replication of avian influenza viruses in humans. *Arch. Virol.*, 119: 37–42.

Capua, I. and Alexander, D.J. (2002). Avian influenza and human health. *Acta Trop.*, 83 (11): 1–6.

Capua, I. and Alexander, D.J. (2004). Avian influenza: recent developments. *Avian Path.*, 33(4): 393–404.

Capua, I. and Marangon, S. (2006). Control of avian influenza in poultry. *Emer. Infect. Dis.*, 12(9): 1319–1324.

Capua, I., Marangon, S. and Selli, L. (1999). Outbreaks of HPAI (H5N2) in Italy during Oct–1997 to Jan. 1998. *Avian Path.*, 28: 455–460.

Cardona, C. (2004). *Avian influenza: biosecurity measures.* Fact sheet 148, University of California Davis.

Chen, Z. (2004). Influenza DNA vaccine: an update. *Chinese Med. J.*, 117(1): 125–132.

Davison, S., Ziegler, A.F. and Eckroade, R.J. (1998). Comparison of an antigen–capture enzyme immunoassay with virus isolation for avian influenza from field samples. *Avian Dis.*, 42(4): 791–795.

Dela Barrera, C.A. and Teran, R.G. (2005). Influenza: forcast for a pandemic. *Aech. Ed. Res.*, 36(6): 628–636.

Fleming, D. (2005). Influenza pandemics and avian flu. *British Med. J.*, 331: 1066–1069.

Hafez, H.M. (2003). Fowl plaque: an old disease that is a continuing danger to poultry. *Tier. Umsch.*, 58(7): 343–351.

Hatta, M. *et al.*, (2001). Molecular basis for high virulence of Hong Kong H5N1 influenza A viruses. *Science*, 293: 1840–42.

Hinshaw, V.S. *et al.* (1981). Replication of avian influenza A viruses in mammals. *Infect. Immun.*, 34: 354–361.

Hoffmann, E. *et al.* (2001). Universal primer set for the full–length amplification of all influenza A viruses. *Arch. Virol.*, 146: 2275–2289.

Horimoto, T. and Kawaoka, Y. (2001). Pandemic threat posed by avian influenza A viruses. *Clin. Microbiol. Rev.*, 14(1): 129–149.

Horimoto, T. and Kawaoka, Y. (2005). Influenza: lesions from past pandemics, warning from current incidents. *Nat. Rev. Microbiol.*, 3(8): 591–600.

Hulse, D.J. *et al.* (2005). Role of domestic ducks in the propagation and biological evolution of highly pathogenic H5N1 influenza viruses in Asia. *Proc. Natl. Acad. Sci.*, USA, 102(30): 10682–10687.

Katx, J.M. (2003). The impact of avian influenza on public health. *Avian Disease*, 47: 914–920.

Kuiken, T. *et al.* (2004). Avian H5N1 influenza in cats. *Science*, 306: 241.

Lee, C.W. and Suarez, D.L. (2005). Avian influenza virus: prospects for prevention and control by vaccination. *Anim. Hlth. Res. Rev.*, 6(1): 1–15.

Lee, C.W. and Suarez, D.L. (2005). Avian influenza virus: prospects for prevention and control by vaccination. *Anim. Hlth Res. Rev.*, 6: 1–15.

Li, K.S. *et al.*, (2004). Genesis of a highly pathogenic and potentially pandemic H5N1 influenza virus in eastern Asia. *Nature*, 430: 209–213.

Liu, J., Xiao, H., Lei, F., Wang, J. And Gao, G.F. (2005). Highly pathogenic H5N1 influenza virus infection in migratory birds. *Science*, 309: 1206–1209.

Mermel, L.A. (2005). Pandemic avian influenza. *Lancet Infect. Dis.*, 5(11): 666–667.

Mo, I.P., Brugh, M. and Fletcher, O.J. (1997). Comparative pathology of chickens experimentally inoculated with avian influenza viruses of low and high pathogenicity. *Avian Dis.*, 41: 125–136.

Monto, A.S. (2005). The threat of an avian influenza pandemic. *N. Engl. J. Med.*, 27: 352(4): 323–324.

Neumann, G., Hatta, M. and Kawaoka, Y. (2003). Reverse genetics for the control of avian influenza. *Avian. Dis.*, 47: 882–887.

Normile, D. (2005). Avian influenza: Europe scrambles to control deadly H5N1 strain. *Science*, 21: 411–420.

Padhi, S., Panigrathi, P.K., Mahapatra, A. and Mahapatra, S. (2004). Avian influenza A (H5N1): a preliminary review. *Indian J. Medical Microbiol.*, 22(3): 143–146.

Paniker, C.K.J. *et al.* (1972). Experimental infection of animals with influenza virus types A and B. *Bull World Health Organization*, 47: 461–463.

Pearson, J.E. (2003). International standards for the control of avian influenza. *Avian Dis.*, 47: 972–975.

Perdue, M.L. and Swayne, D.E. (2005). Public health risk from avian influenza viruses. *Avian Disease*, 49(3): 317–327.

Perdue, M.L., Suarez, D. L. and Swayne, D.E. (1999). Avian influenza in the 1990s. *Poultry and Avian Biology Reviews*, 11: 1–20.

Permin, A. (2004). Avian influenza is spreading. Now avian influenza is also in pigs. *Dan. Vet.*, 87(19): 10–11.

Poddar, S.K. (2002). Influenza virus types and subtypes detection by single step single tube multiplex RT–PCR and agarose gel electrophoresis. *J. Virol Meth.*, 99: 63–70.

Pollack, C.V., Kam, C.W. and Mak, Y.K. (1998). Update: isolation of avian influenza A (H5N1) viruses from human beings–Hong Kong 1997–1998. *Ann. Emer. Med.*, 31(5): 647–649.

Reid, A.H. and Taubenberger, J.K. (1999). The 1918 flu and other influenza pandemics: over there and back again. *Lab. Invest.*, 79(2): 95–101.

Rimmelzwann, G.F. *et al.* (2001). Pathogenesis of influenza A (H5N1) virus infection in a primate model. *J. Virol.*, 75: 6687–91.

Rogers, G.N. and D'Souza, B.L. (1989). Receptor binding properties of human and animal H1 influenza virus isolates. *Virol.*, 173: 317–322.

Shortridge, K.F. (1999). Poultry and the influenza H5N1 outbreak in Hong Kong, 1997: abridged chronology and virus isolation. *Vaccine*, 17: 526–529.

Shortridge, K.F., Peiris, J.S.M. and Guan, Y. (2003). The next influenza pandemic: lesions from Hong Kong. *Soc. Appl. Microbiol. Sym. Series*, 32: 70–79.

Smith, G.J., Fan, X.H. and Wang, J. (2006). Emergence and predominance of an H5N1 influenza variant in China. *PNAS*, 103(45): 16936–16941.

Stallknecht, D.E. and Shane, S.M. (1988). Host range of avian influenza virus in free living birds. *Vet. Res. Comm.*, 12: 125–141.

Starick, E. and Werner, O. (2003). Detection of H7 avian influenza virus directly from poultry specimens. *Avian Dis.*, 47: 1187–1189.

Suarez, D.L. (1998). Comparison of highly virulent H5N1 influenza A viruses isolated from humans and chickens in Hong Kong. *J. Virol.*, 72: 6678–6688.

Suarez, D.L. and Schultz, C.S. (2000). Immunology of avian influenza virus: a review. *Dev. Comp. Immunol.*, 24: 269–283.

Suarez, D.L.(2000). Evolution of avian influenza viruses. *Vet. Microbiol.*, 74: 15–27.

Suarez, D.L., Perdue, M.L., Cox, N., Rowe, T. and Swayne, D.E. (1998). Comparison of highly virulent H5N1 influenza viruses isolated from humans and chickens from Hong Kong. *J. Virol.*, 72: 6678–6688.

Sugimura, T., Murakami, Y. and Ogawa, T. (2000). The susceptibility of cultured cells to avian influenza viruses. *J. Vet. Med. Sci.*, 62(6): 659–660.

Swayne, D.E. (2000). Understanding the ecology and epidemiology of avian influenza viruses: implications for zoonotic potential. In: *Emerging Diseases of Animals*, Brown, C.C. and Bolin, C.A. (eds.) ASM Press, Washington, D.C., pp 101–130.

Swayne, D.E. and Suarez, D.L. (2000). Highly pathogenic avian influenza. *Rev. Sci. Tech. Off. Int. Epiz.*, 19: 463–482.

Swayne, D.E., Beck, J.R., Garcia, M., Stone, H.D. (1999). Influence of virus strain and antigen mass on efficacy of H5 avian influenza inactivated vaccines. *Avian Path.*, 28: 245–255.

Swayne, D.E., Beck, J.R., Perdue, M.L. and Beard, C.W. (2001). Efficacy of vaccines in chickens against highly pathogenic Hong Kong H5N1 avian influenza. *Avian. Dis.*, 45(2): 355–365.

Tam, J.S. (2002). Influenza A (H5N1) in Hong Kong: an overview. *Vaccine*, 15(20): Suppl.2: S77–81.

Thornley, M. (2004). Avian influenza ravages Thai tigers. *Aus. Vet. J.*, 82(11): 652–655.

Tumpey, T.M., Alvarez, R., Swayne, D.E. and Suarez, D.L. (2005). Diagnostic approach for differentiating infected from vaccinated poultry on the basis of antibodies to NS1, the non-structural protein of influenza A virus. *J. Clin. Microbiol.*, 43(2): 676–683.

Villarreal-Chavez, C. and Rivera-Cruz, E. (2003). An update on avian influenza in Mexico. *Avian Dis.*, 47: 1002–1005.

Wan, X.F., Ren, T., Luo, K.J., Liao, M., Zhang, G.H., Xu, D. and Xin, C.A. (2005). Genetic characterization of H5N1 avian influenza viruses isolated in Southern China during the 2003–04 avian influenza outbreaks. *Arch. Virol.*, 150 (6): 1257–1266.

Webby, R.J., Perez, D.R., Coleman, J.S., Guan, Y. and Wester, R.G. (2004). Responsive to a pandemic alert: use of reverse genetics for rapid development of influenza vaccines. *Lancet*, 363: 1099–1103.

Webster, R.G. and Hulse, D.J. (2004). Microbial adaptation and change: avian influenza. *Rev. Sci. Tech.*, 23(2): 453–465.

Webster, R.G., Bean, W. J., Gorman, O.T. and Kawaoka, Y. (1992). Evolution and ecology of influenza A viruses. *Microbiol. Rev.*, 56: 152–179.

Webster, R.G., Guan, Y., Poon, L., Webby, R. and Peiris, M. (2005). The spread of the H5N1 bird flu epidemic in Asia in 2004. *Arch. Virol. Suppl.*, 19: 117–129.

Winkel, G. (1997). Biosecurity in poultry production. *Acta Vet. Hungarica,* 45(3): 361–372.

Yuen, K. Y., Chan, P.K.S., Peiris, M. and Cheng, A.F.B. (1998). Clinical features and rapid viral diagnosis of human disease associated with avian influenza A H5N1 virus. *Lancet*, 351: 467–471.

Yuen, K.Y. and Wong, S.S. (2005). Human infection by avian influenza A H5N1. *Hong Kong Med. J.*, 11(3): 189–199.

Yuen, K.Y., Chan, P.K.S., Peiris, M., Tsang, D.N.C. and Cheng, A.F.B. (1998). Clinical features and rapid viral viral diagnosis of human disease associated with avian influenza A H5N1 virus. *Lancet*, 351: 467–471.

Zhou, E., Chan, M., Hecket, R.A., Riva, J. and Cantin, M.F. (1998). Evaluation of a competitive ELISA for detection of antibodies against avian influenza virus nucleoprotein. *Avian Dis.*, 42: 517–522.

Index